Psychological Medicine

Trevor H. Turner

A diagnostic analysis of the Casebooks of Ticehurst House Asylum, 1845–1890

MONOGRAPH SUPPLEMENT 21

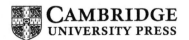

CAMBRIDGE UNIVERSITY PRESS
Cambridge, New York, Melbourne, Madrid, Cape Town,
Singapore, São Paulo, Delhi, Tokyo, Mexico City

Cambridge University Press
The Edinburgh Building, Cambridge CB2 8RU, UK

Published in the United States of America by
Cambridge University Press, New York

www.cambridge.org
Information on this title: www.cambridge.org/9780521429863

First published 1992

A catalogue record for this publication is available from the British Library

ISBN 978-0-521-42986-3 Paperback

CONTENTS

This work, based on an M.D. thesis submitted to the University of London, was only made possible by the continued support, encouragement and assistance, both material and personal, of the staff at the Wellcome Institute for the History of Medicine in London. In particular I am grateful to Dr William Bynum for his invaluable advice, his close reading of the provisional manuscript, and his overall supervision of my prolonged period of research. I am also indebted to Charlotte MacKenzie for details of Ticehurst House, to Julia Sheppard for help with the archives, to Michael Neve for his patient and stimulating forbearance of my presence in his office, and to Andrew Foley for his 'oriental' understanding of my photocopying needs. The typescript relied on the brilliant professionalism of Sally Bragg, to whom my gratitude is unbounded.

    I am also most grateful to Dr D. E. Allen of the Wellcome Trust for providing research expenses, and to the Wellcome Unit as a whole for material help in the library, photocopying, and with archives.

    The support of my wife and family has of course been of the essence in completing the project.

LIST OF TABLES

SYNOPSIS Ticehurst House, a private asylum, flourished during the nineteenth century as the most expensive of such establishments, being owned and run by the Drs Newington over five successive generations. The discovery of the full set of patient casebooks begun in 1845–6 made it possible to review in detail the clinical features of a complete cohort of patients admitted to the asylum between 1845 and 1890. Six-hundred-and-one patients were thus analysed in terms of their age, sex, length of stay, symptoms, treatment and outcome. Modern operational diagnoses were used, and 80% of the cohort were found to conform to Research Diagnostic Criteria, in particular to the categories for schizophrenia and manic-depressive disorder. An additional finding was the high prevalence of movement and postural disorder among the schizophrenic group, as well as a significant trend towards the selection of a treatable, good-outcome group of patients with manic-depressive illness. These results are discussed by comparison with other modern studies of the asylum period, and in the contemporary context of Victorian psychological medicine. It is suggested that the violence, physicality and chronicity of psychotic illness must be seen as central to the debate about the rise of the asylum in nineteenth-century Britain. Furthermore, the similarity in core symptoms found in such patients and those seen in the 1980s indicates that the categories 'schizophrenia' and 'manic-depressive disorder' have a robust validity that is not confined to the social parameters of a particular time period.

Address for correspondence: Dr Trevor H. Turner, Department of Psychological Medicine, St Bartholomew's Hospital, West Smithfield, London EC1A 7BE.

Introduction

'The history of psychiatry is essentially the history of humanism.'

(Zilboorg & Henry, 1941 p. 524.)

'The science of mental disease, as it would develop in the asylum, would always be only of the order of observation and classification. It would not be a dialogue.'

(Foucault, 1967, p. 250.)

'The new historiography insistently poses the question: Is there any such natural object as "madness" at all?'

(Bynum et al. 1985.)

The transformation of the history of psychiatry into the history of 'madness' has been a useful product of the anti-psychiatry movement. It is now customary to view traditional historians (e.g. Zilboorg & Henry, 1941; Leigh, 1961; Alexander & Selesnick, 1966) as presenting a 'whig' view of progress and to discount the role of medical practitioners in exploring their own past. This predominance of the perspective of social history was exemplified by the minimal medical representation in the 1985 'report from the front line', *The Anatomy of Madness* (vols. I and II, Bynum et al. 1985). But the introductions to these volumes did provide succinct and rich summaries of both versions of historical analysis, taking a more neutral stance. While Foucault is still seen as the major influence against the modern meliorist school, Andrew Scull in his *Museums of Madness* (1979), has probably had the more persistent effect. Notwithstanding the admirably researched work of Parry-Jones (1972) or Hunter & MacAlpine (1963, 1974), there has been (amid the professional data, primary sources and publicized monographs), little space for the psychiatric clinicians to add significantly to the historical account. Which is not to say that they have been suppressed; rather that their medical bias has been ignored amid the rich discoveries of social archaeology.

This process, of peering into the business of treating mental illness, reflects the recurring fascination of madness down the ages, as well as the present practical debate about 'community care'. This latter phrase has become so over-used that the present Chief Medical Officer felt constrained to ask for clarification as to its meaning (Acheson, 1985). In essence, though, it can be seen historically as the response to the waning 'Asylum Era', wherein the buildings used to house the mentally ill have become stigmatized as part of the problem. Now that they are starting to fall down, the asylums are being classified as a dreadful mistake, as a means of removing an innocently deviant population from the public eye, as a form of social control, as anti-therapeutic. 'It seems likely that the dread of mental illness may be nothing more than a dread of what happened to the mentally ill, the symbol of which is the asylum' (Kosky, 1986). While there seems little doubt that the moral therapy, trumpeted by Tuke (1813), gradually ossified into what might better be termed architectural, or even structural, therapy, and concern about asylum care was apparent within a generation of the 1845 'Asylums' Act, there has nevertheless been little detailed research into the possible medical reasons behind this shift. Why did these institutions continue to flourish? Why did the asylums become enormous, unwieldy monstrosities, piling up their chronic 'incurables' despite repeated concern. Given a late-Victorian atmosphere (exemplified by the response to Charles Reade's 1863 *Hard Cash* and the 1877 Select Committee enquiry into lunacy certification) of doubts about alienists; given an 1890 Lunacy Act aimed at a legalistic control of the certification process so as to make it more difficult to commit someone to an asylum; given the low esteem of the psychiatric profession in contrast to that of other medical specialities, why did more and more citizens find themselves placed in asylums? In bald terms, why did the numbers of certified insane increase by 255·1% between 1859 and 1910, while the population increased by 83·7%? (*Lunacy in England and Wales*, 1910).

The social explanation of those figures has been outlined by Scull (1979), and a similar rationale underlies the modern-day community-care movement. This perspective is profoundly sceptical of an overarching incarceration of those deemed mentally ill. Sceptical also of the boundaries of psychiatric diagnosis, it prefers to elaborate the political, industrial and cultural context, wherein the 'recognition and interpretation of mental illness, indeed its whole meaning, are culture-bound and change profoundly from epoch to epoch, in ways inexplicable' (Bynum *et al.* 1985). The demise of the asylums is thus seen as representing the exposure of psychiatry to its own shortcomings. Institutionalization created its own 'institutional neurosis' (Barton, 1976), and the opening of the door to care in the community could be seen as the first step in examining the 'myth of mental illness' (Szasz, 1972). The urge to de-medicalize behaviour that might have a moral and social basis, and the powerful gurus representing these ideas, have grasped the public and political imagination. Such analyses may even shade into more extreme views based on the 'social construction of illness', wherein the reality of psychiatric disease is itself questioned. For example, Scheff (1966, p. 25) has suggested 'psychiatric symptoms are...labelled violations of social norms', and only arise in a 'particular society'.

Modern research, as exemplified by the collected papers in *The Anatomy of Madness* (Bynum *et al.* 1985, 1988) has partially blunted this crusade by insisting on a more detailed filling in of the picture. The economic aspects of asylums have yet to be properly examined, and it is clear that 'psychiatry actually made progress as a discipline during the 19th century' (Bynum *et al.* 1985). Social control theory may be enticing but does it fully explain the particular use of doctors, mental illness, and evangelical reform as a *modus operandi*? It does not seem even to attempt to grasp the sheer violence, helplessness and social vulnerability of those felt, in the layperson's view, to be insane. Colaizzi (1989) quotes from the *Virginia Gazette* of 1769 on a domestic murder: 'It is really shocking to see the number of miserable people who have lost the use of their reason, that are daily wandering about, for want of a proper house to keep them confined in. If there had been such a place, this poor man would not have met with the above

untimely end' (p. 11). Such sentiments are expressed, almost verbatim, in the modern press, and recent in-depth studies of nineteenth-century asylum care (e.g. Finnane, 1981; Tomes, 1984; Digby, 1984; Dwyer, 1987; Garton, 1988) have detailed the difficulties of organizing, staffing and protecting institutions for the care of stigmatized, unpredictable, 'mad folk'. In the words of one (Dwyer, 1987, p. 216), 'asylum doctors were expected to act in accordance with sometimes amorphous, often contradictory, and always forceful social dictates, even when they were not given the means with which to satisfy society's complex demands'.

Alternative theories have been put forward by Torrey and Hare, based on a disease model. In *Schizophrenia and Civilization* (1980) the former elaborated the notion of a 'new' illness, arising in the nineteenth century, since 'the epidemiology of schizophrenia strongly supports an association between the disease and civilization' (p. 187). He argued that this association was likely to be causal and 'the most likely causes are biological'. The evidence he adduced included seasonality of birth (more schizophrenics are born in winter months), the increased prevalence of schizophrenia in urban populations, its apparent rarity before 1800 and the lack of data to support the various psychosocial theories. The likely causative agent he regarded as a virus (or viruses) interacting with a genetic predisposition. Using an epidemiological perspective, Hare has elaborated upon this theory, suggesting that there may well have been a true increase in insanity during the nineteenth century (Hare, 1983). Admitting that the 'idea of schizophrenia (or a common type of it) being a recent disease is still only tentative', he nevertheless felt that such a theory could 'account for many aspects of the history of schizophrenia' (1986). His fully developed 'recency hypothesis' (1988) focused on 'adolescent insanity' in particular. As a parallel model, he has also pointed to the considerable evidence, both contemporary and modern, that General Paralysis of the Insane (GPI) increased significantly during the nineteenth century in industrialized Europe (Hare, 1959). While urbanization or toxic agents may have promoted such disease prevalence, the general approach of this school of thought is clear. The asylums were, in a large part, a response to a new range of chronic brain diseases presenting with mental symptoms and brought on by the various accompaniments of civilization.

Critics of this view (e.g. Jeste *et al.* 1985) can be found in several areas. Many retrospective diagnosticians would insist that schizophrenic symptoms are perfectly visible in the older historical records if one knows where to look. From Edgar's feigned Tom O'Bedlam in Shakespeare's *King Lear*, from the lives of the saints and other religious figures, from the records of St Bartholomew's Hospital, there is variably good evidence of behaviour and symptoms that fit modern diagnostic systems, such as DSM-III (APA, 1980). In a recent summary of this approach, Jeste *et al.* (1985) admit there is 'no definitive answer' but insist that 'schizophrenia is probably very old'. An alternative critique from Scull (1984) has suggested the likelihood of a more socio-cultural explanation. Once asylums are available there is a lowering of the threshold tolerating abnormal behaviour. Increasingly mild cases are thus disposed of by their relatives and the asylum doctors cooperate in this process because of their need to expand their influence and professional roles. The apparent increase in insanity thus reflects a conspiracy to hive off the economically burdensome and socially deviant (and embarrassing) members of one's family. Allied to these approaches is the undoubted fact that increasing diagnostic perspicacity accompanies specialization within medicine. Once behaviour, perhaps formerly seen as eccentric, silly, but harmless, is defined as an illness, then more individuals are labelled as 'mad' without there being any true increase in the numbers of that category in a given society. Diagnostic insights (e.g. Legionnaire's disease) inevitably lead to the perception of an increased disease incidence, whether or not a true increase is taking place.

Of course, such criticisms of the 'disease theory' are not coherent among themselves. Diagnostic methods would be queried by Scull and Foucault, who viewed the search for professional power despite a lack of diagnostic (or therapeutic) expertise as the driving force of asylum expansion. The notion that a serious mental illness, today termed 'schizophrenia', has been plaguing humanity throughout history regardless of cultures, customs or life-events, would likewise be disowned by the social constructionist school (e.g. Scheff, 1966). Nor is such fragmentation confined to the historical debate. The first asylum closure (in Britain) has now taken place (Banstead – October 1986) amid a confusion of voices. The mainstream and government line welcomes this advance towards care in the community. Researchers point to increased therapeutic potency, economics, and the need to destigmatize mental illness as underlying this change. Critics cite the expansion in prison places and the increase in vagrancy as evidence of its wrongfulness (see Turner, 1985). The gap, between denouncing asylums as social constructs and praising them as medical achievements, refuses to close. That the modern-day and historical debates parallel each other so closely indicates just how central is this issue to our understanding of the recent history of 'madness', as exemplified by Andrew Scull's work on decarceration (1977).

But while explorations into the social history of those deemed mad can only enrich our understanding and treatment of them today, it is important to define terms. Little attempt is made, among historians, to differentiate between gross psychosis, overt brain disease, abnormalities of personality and minor mood changes in even the best summaries or papers of today. Thus, Porter, in his introduction to the *Anatomy of Madness*, vol. 1 (1985), praises the Victorians for 'bringing order, clarity and universality to the basic concepts, indeed the very language of psychopathological practice', while nowhere delimiting his use of the term 'madness'. Scull (1979) concentrated on 'deviant behaviour' and used other linguistic devices that have been aptly criticized for their implicit assumptions (Jones, 1982). Rothman (*The Discovery of the Asylum*, 1971) was more circumspect, asking 'are reason and unreason mutually exclusive?' in his analysis of the Foucaultian position. Anne Digby (1985) entitled her detailed and sober description of The York Retreat, *Madness, Morality and Medicine*, but was careful in her terms and confined herself to contemporary diagnostic language.

From the medical viewpoint the excessive repetition of one term, such as 'madness', to embrace a wide range of behaviours, disorders, diagnoses (and their courses and consequences) is loose and unhelpful. While it may reflect contemporary custom and help to link the attitudes and theories of different times, such generalization fails to delineate the nitty-gritty requirements of a suitable response or even treatment. If we wish to understand why asylums were built, it is not enough to regard their inmates merely as versions of a unitary analysis. Such an extraordinary commitment of finance, professional time, and legal and administrative resources demands a more detailed dissection of the meaning of insanity. The fashionable 'hypochondria' of George Cheyne (1733) had little to do with the ravings of a brain-damaged epileptic. Whereas the first could (it seems) respond to ingenious insights and intelligent, verbalized, concern, the other demands a patience and physical forbearance (in the face of dirt, violence and stupidity) that may be both demeaning and intolerable. Such a differentiated understanding of varieties of mental illness has been masked, even in modern times, by terms such as 'institutional neurosis' which are said to describe the chronic asylum inmate. Russell Barton (1976), Wing & Brown (1970) and Goffman (1961) have elaborated upon this theme from several viewpoints, but modern work has found similar deficits in cognition and behaviour in non-institutionalized patients (Johnstone _et al._ 1981). This is not to deny the effects of institutions, but rather to assert the primacy of illness in creating such abnormalities.

The question thus arises as to how possible it is clearly to characterize the Victorian asylum patient. Not because of a meliorist need to display the progress of modern psychiatry in making diagnoses, nor in a belief that such an understanding is the key to unlocking the mystery of asylumization. The forces of economic and industrial change (cf. Cooper & Sartorius, 1977) and the powerful religious motives of the times are probably far more significant in deciding the form of the therapeutic response. If, however, we take as a hypothesis the notion that mental illness is primarily a cultural construct, with symptoms and course largely dependent on the attitudes and conditions of its times, we can attempt to find out – given the contemporary notes describing patients' behaviour – whether similar 'illnesses' exist today. The clear recognition of psychopathology indistinguishable from modern versions of psychiatric diagnosis would disprove our hypothesis, and strengthen the validity of the medical model in its broadest nosological sense. This process of retrospective diagnosis certainly has its limits but has been widely used in a variety of contexts with useful results (e.g. Klaf & Hamilton, 1961; Tsuang & Winokur, 1975).

A particular example, relevant to this study, is that of Shepherd (1957). Examining records from an English county asylum for the two triennia 1931–3 and 1945–7, he was able to extract factual information (e.g. sex, age, dates of admission and discharge) without difficulty while acknowledging the more 'equivocal' data of diagnosis and length of history. Stating clearly that 'the difficulties inherent in psychiatric diagnosis confront all workers in this field', he found notes summarized, an 'economy of observation' and a problematical system of classification. Using all available records, notes and letters, he was nevertheless able to focus 'on the outstanding psychiatric feature during the period of medical observation' and employed a broad triple classification: functional psychoses; psychoses associated with organic and senile diseases; and miscellaneous disorders. This was not dissimilar to that chosen for this study (see below, Method section), and enabled him to demonstrate a large increase in admissions and turnover rate, related to a diagnosis of affective disorder, while his schizophrenic group was largely unchanged. This relationship between diagnosis and the 'consequent functional transformation' of the mental hospital was significant, reflected 'legislative and administrative measures' and seemed relevant to the wider national scene. The simple centrality of diagnosis in discussing asylum practices cannot therefore be ignored amid the welter of social data or explanations, and it can be formulated as an independent variable in clear language.

With regard to Victorian patients, the ability to perform such an analysis has been limited by the lack of notes sufficiently detailed to provide appropriate data. Robinson (1988), however, has used the detailed 1880–9 casebooks of the Crichton Royal Institution in Scotland to compare delusional depressive illness then and now, showing a greater prevalence for severe (delusional) conditions in the nineteenth-century admissions. There was no difficulty in fitting nineteenth-century descriptions into modern categories, although some might suggest that there is no true cultural difference between Victorian and modern Britain, that they are part of the same era and share the same social construction. Others would reject the extrapolation of one asylum's notes to the whole asylum world, particularly if that asylum was private and exclusive. Others would view the whole notion of retrospective diagnosis as 'presentist' and historically unhelpful, since our understanding of the role of psychiatric diagnosis in Victorian asylums will not be enhanced by the banal statement that patients were 'schizophrenic' or had 'Alzheimer's disease'. While it may benefit the modern clinician to have descriptions of the course of illnesses unaffected by modern drugs, modern conditions or the selective bias of the textbook author, how can modern labels clarify our understanding of past practices?

There seem to be at least two possible answers to this question, aside from the obvious point that historians and psychiatrists search the records of history from different academic and experimental viewpoints, the one seeking primarily to understand the past, the other seeking also to understand a professional present. First, the use of modern diagnoses can be seen as a form of translation, in the way that the decipherment of linear B from Ancient Crete gave valuable information as to the historical roots of the Greek language. This translation, of Victorian casenotes, may likewise clarify the causes, courses and diagnostic language of the times. Secondly, the clear description of recognizable disease entities enables us to review epidemiological data from the past as Torrey (1980) and Hare (1983) have done, so as to generate or disprove hypotheses about the natural history of many ill-understood conditions. Were it to be clearly shown that schizophrenia-like illnesses increased dramatically throughout the nineteenth century, as opposed to other forms of psychosis, this knowledge might help to clarify some of the causes operating in the rise of the asylums – not as an explanation, nor as a moral judgement, but as a means of obtaining insights into the Victorian reaction to mental illness, whether at the professional, personal or social level. Such answers do not, of course, directly oppose the arguments of those who deny the reality of psychiatric illness. But they do provide the foundations for a coherent historical understanding of the nature of such disorders, across time and place.

The purpose of this study must then be seen as intensive rather than extensive, focusing on a small collection of primary sources despite the broad historical themes outlined above. It attempts to portray the medical details of Ticehurst Asylum, in East Sussex, between 1845 and 1890, using the casebooks serendipitously rescued from the cellars in the late 1970s. These are complete for the period in question, as are the admission and discharge registers, medical visitation books and numerous other administrative records (see Method section).

The first question addressed was the possibility of extracting sufficient details of behaviour and psychopathology so as to reach a reasonably firm diagnosis. Once a preliminary survey had shown that this was likely (see Method section), the question arose as to what use could be made of such knowledge. Of course, a negative response to the first question could have arisen for several reasons. It might have been that the notes were simply too sparse to allow of any detailed analysis. This has been a major problem for clinicians in applying their diagnostic efforts to other records of the past, although rich individual studies of isolated works have been made. Kroll & Bachrach (1982) have reviewed the medieval chronicles to show that mental illness and its treatment in those times bears comparison with modern approaches. Hunter & MacAlpine (1963), in their magisterial collection of primary sources, provide numerous examples of detailed psychopathology and constantly insist on the appropriateness of a modern diagnostic label. The standard histories (e.g. Zilboorg & Henry, 1941) include anecdotes and written 'cases' exemplifying recognizable signs and symptoms. But while these may be interesting to psychiatrists, they derive from a random collection of sources and do not enable us to take a consistent, historical view of the phenomena. Furthermore, they can lead to unreliable flights of fancy as portrayed in *Schizophrenia 1677* (1956), wherein MacAlpine and Hunter took Freud to task for his psychoanalytic theorizing over a case of demoniacal possession. While forcefully debunking the 'repressed homosexuality' theory of psychosis, as derived by Freud from this and the Schreber case, on the grounds that it was apparently replete with logical lacunae, Hunter & Mac-Alpine themselves seem to have become enmeshed by Freud's inconsistencies.

For the case of Christopher Haizmann is given in excellent detail in their monograph, making it possible to review the symptoms in the light of modern Research Diagnostic Criteria (RDC) as used in this analysis of the Ticehurst House records. The RDC (Spitzer *et al.* 1975) lay down certain operational criteria concerning schizophrenia as a diagnosis, insisting on a certain time-course (2 weeks) of active symptoms, a specific range of symptoms (e.g. third-person auditory hallucinations) and the exclusion of features related to manic-depressive or organic pathology. Yet the episodic course of this 1677 case, the strongly visual nature of the hallucinations, the alterations in mood and level of conscious awareness, all point much more towards some form of temporal-lobe epilepsy or even manic-depressive illness. Although colourful and well documented, this is just the type of case that represents too many exceptional and unusual features – thus perhaps its survival in the records? – to be used as evidence for a persisting and common diagnostic category.

By contrast, the problem of insufficiently detailed notes is particularly apparent in viewing the records of Bethlem Hospital, the archives of which would seem an obvious source of diagnostic plunder. But whether one takes the cases recorded by Haslam in his *Observations on Insanity* (1798), or looks through the nineteenth-century casebooks, the lack of persistent data is striking. While the demography and practices of the hospital can be closely followed, and the truth behind 'Bedlam' appropriately reviewed (cf. Allderidge, 1985), it is not possible to apply, for example, RDC with any consistency because there is simply not enough detail recorded.

In a random review of the Bethlem Casebooks from 1846 to 1885 the sparseness of information could be attributed to several factors. In 1846, when Dr E. T. Monro (1790–1856) was physician, two pages were allotted per patient, including a standard format sheet with headings, as 'Supposed Cause of Insanity' and 'Temper and Disposition Prior to Insanity Commencing', which was usually filled in briefly. However, the medical notes then rarely extend beyond a quarter of a page from the date of admission,

and contain little more than a diagnosis and behavioural description. Only six out of forty-two patients had a 'statement of the Medical Attendant' actually filled in. Between 18 September and 25 December Monro described twenty-six patients as having 'melancholia', five each with 'mania' and 'monomania', three as 'flighty', and one each as 'polymania' and 'religious excitement' (one was not diagnosed). By 1855 there are four pages allotted to each patient but only about one sixth of the space available is used for notes. These consist of the recent or past history – often written three to four weeks after admission – and the briefest of reports every one or two months, such as 'No change' or 'No Improvement', etc. No diagnoses are apparent and the impression is of small islands of notes in a sea of blank paper. By 1865 there is a little more detail in the medical certificates and an occasional diagnosis, but the written notes rarely exceed one page. By 1875 there is a distinct improvement, the notes extending to two half-pages, and death certificates (GPI is prominent) are included. There are occasional letters and newspaper reports, and printed headings (e.g. 'Family History', 'Habits', 'Tendency to leave home', 'Hallucinations?') are found in the first half-page of the medical notes to ensure that something appropriate is actually recorded by the medical officer. By 1885 there is little extra apart from the extension of the printed headings to include findings 'On Admission'. Comments are required on 'Sleep', 'Dreams', 'Walk', 'Reflexes', 'Weight', 'Handwriting' and 'Dynanometer'. However, this section is usually not filled in, and poorly done when attempted. Diagnoses are uncommon, it is rare for more than one page of notes to be recorded, and the most useful source of information is found in the attached letters of relatives and friends. One patient's father describes 'voices', 'extreme indolence and obstinacy', 'great irritability', 'peculiarities of dress' and 'whims about food', a plethora of observations that are by contrast absent from the medical notes.

Bethlem was in the main confined to taking people for no more than one year, so the course of chronic illness could not anyway be followed. Nevertheless, the sparseness of detail is clearly unsuitable for any attempt at retrospective diagnosis and the notes of many other public asylums are similarly limited, in my own experience.

As stated above though, the Ticehurst notes may have been unsuitable for another reason, namely the data contained in them might not have conformed to any modern constellations of symptoms or diagnostic labels. The language, behaviour and outcomes may have been entirely strange, outside our present notions of mental illness. All the patients might have been described as speaking in tongues, as standing on their heads, as demanding to see their lawyers in clear logical language. While many variegated symptoms might have been elicited, however, the patterns should largely have conformed to those seen today if the beginnings of a retrospective diagnosis were to be considered.

Given, then, that reaching a diagnosis was possible, how might this process add information to that available as part of the usual record? One answer might lie in the details of the age, sex, marital status and personal background of the patients. These were routinely given, as were the dates of admission and discharge and the contemporary diagnostic label. The social topography of mental illness, an understanding of the language used to describe it and the methods of treatment might be clarified in the light of modern diagnosis. There are, of course, problems in using casenotes of this type, as Digby (1985) discusses in the appendix to her monograph on The Retreat. Admitting them to be a 'neglected but rich source', she warns that 'they raise difficult problems of interpretation, including the central issue of how far the historian can generalize from a particular sample'. She appends four detailed case-histories so as to illustrate 'changing methods of treatment and distinctive attitudes to Retreat patients during the nineteenth century'. She warns against taking The Retreat, with its small size and selected, private clientele, as a model for the large public asylums, although its 'impact on the general climate of opinion' is likely to have been greater than the confines of documentary evidence. Likewise Dwyer (1987) regarded the casebooks of the Utica and Willard asylums in nineteenth-century New York as the 'richest and most difficult to interpret' of her sources, offering as they did 'tantalizing glimpses of

patients' pre-institutional lives' as well as details of 'behaviour and treatment'. But she also warned that 'they entice the twentieth-century reader into conjectures about the relationship between asylums and the communities they served' (p. 5).

Such strictures would also apply to Ticehurst, although a regular intercourse between public and private asylums would broaden the importance of an apparently select (in economic terms) clientele. As expressed by Dr J. W. Eastwood (1863), in his paper on 'Private Asylums for the Insane', while there were differences in the management and social treatment, this was not so in regard to 'the moral and medical treatment of the two classes of patients'. So although it is clear that caution is needed in placing casenote data from a private asylum into the wider historical context, there still seems to be an important role for these sources in providing clues about the nature of insanity in Victorian England. Whether rich patients would have been more seriously disturbed than the neglected poor is a moot point, examined in more detail in the Discussion. Certainly there is no evidence that the core symptoms of psychosis (in terms of their form) vary according to social class, today or in the past; the content of delusions, however, and disturbed behaviour secondary to such symptoms, is naturally related to gender, culture and class origins. From the internal psychiatric viewpoint, therefore, it seemed likely that an unspoilt picture of the courses of mental illness could be obtained from sufficiently detailed notes of the past. As such, this data could provide an historical control sample to set against the outcome of modern patients treated with a range of potent drugs, post-Freudian psychotherapeutic techniques and varying social placements.

A contrasting approach to the study of Victorian asylum life, although based on the same materials, has been the parallel thesis of MacKenzie (1986a), entitled 'A Family Asylum: A History of the Private Madhouse at Ticehurst in Sussex, 1792–1917'. Her work covers a broader time-span, and concentrates designedly on the social context, with an extensive outline of the Newington family. As such it provides not so much an alternative view of events, but rather a 'focus on the relationship between the family and the asylum'. While rejecting much of the analyses of Foucault and Scull, she does not 'see it as the historian's task to make retrospective diagnoses or discuss whether or not asylum inmates were "really" ill'. However, she does wish 'to elaborate the way in which asylum inmates were perceived by their contemporaries and by themselves', and to understand 'how well psychiatry related to prevailing standards and ideals of moral and social behaviour'. While one might suggest that the language of illness and the experiences of the patients are vital to an understanding of contemporary views (as stated earlier in this Introduction), her direct outline of the social matrix shows how differing historical perspectives can be derived from similar source materials. Such approaches are in the main complementary, displaying the power of psychiatry's history to enrich understanding across disciplines.

MacKenzie's conclusions are, however, problematical, in that she has to cover a prolonged time-period, using data of differing details and quality, without any central hypothesis to unite her work. She believes 'psychiatry also has an emancipatory potential', and accepts the role of 'care', as opposed to 'cure' in asylum work. The decline of therapeutic optimism in the last third of the nineteenth century is also a significant theme, which she associates with a 'deterioration in treatment'. Most controversially, she is critical of 'psychiatry's latent moralism', regarding it as a 'fundamentally moral enterprise', and she finds it 'difficult to conceive of a standard for "psychological functions" which would not incorporate some moral values'. Her final comment is to call for 'greater self-questioning within psychiatry of some of the possible human costs (as well as benefits) of a stronger commitment to the biomedical model'. Yet it might well be argued that without a clear definition of the 'biomedical model', and without constructing some form of diagnostic language, attributing moral overtones to writings from the past is all too easy. The false equivalence of the term 'moral insanity' with the modern notion of sociopath or psychopath is an obvious example.

While MacKenzie has provided rich details of the dialogue, economic, familial and educational, around the Newingtons and their asylum, there is a constant sense of a gap in the picture, a failure to grasp the dimensions of the malign experience of psychotic illness.

In summary then, the aim of this study was twofold. Using the uniquely elaborate notes from Ticehurst asylum, it was designed to examine in detail the case-histories of those deemed mentally ill in the second half of the nineteenth century. Apart from the intrinsic value of providing a rich picture of asylum life from the clinical perspective, it is postulated that the information may throw light on the overall developments of the 'Asylum Era' as well as those occurring today, for example under the notion of 'community care'. At a less ambitious, secondary level some of the problems of understanding the symptoms of schizophrenia-like illness (e.g. is dyskinesia intrinsic to the disease process?) and of coping with disturbed behaviour may also benefit from historical insights. To what extent such an approach can usefully aid historical interpretation is more contentious, but the role of diagnosis and the language of Victorian psychopathology have been little explored at this basic level. While the theories of mental illness, the diagnostic schemata of Pinel (1806), Esquirol (1845), Skae (1863), Griesinger (1867), Maudsley (1895), etc., and the developments of psychological science have been regularly assessed (e.g. Lewis, 1934; Berrios, 1984, 1988; Clark, 1981, 1988), there is no direct evidence of the way in which such diagnoses were used by practising alienists. In essence therefore this work is part of 'the labour of actually finding out', since we remain ignorant of much of what went on, at ward level, in nineteenth-century asylums. While agreeing with Rothman (1971, p. xx) that 'we are duty bound to move back and forth, in and out' of the asylum, there does seem a need (despite the work of Finnane, 1981; Tomes, 1984; Digby, 1985; Dwyer, 1987, and others) for more inside information.

Method

The basic resource for the study was the collection of records transferred from Ticehurst House, Sussex, to the Wellcome Institute in October 1980. These had been discovered in the basement of the present building, during a general survey of the house when it came under the control of new management. From the clinical point of view, the Casebooks were the most remarkable find, in that their consistency and detail over a long period of time (1846–1917) probably have no equal in contemporary archives. Supplemented by the Admission Registers and the Registers of Removal, Discharge and Deaths, they provide a continuous record of the medical management of patients from admission to discharge or death, sometime supplemented by relatives' letters, patients' letters and drawings, letters of visiting physicians, newspaper cuttings, details of previous and subsequent history and post-mortem records. There are also books recording the use of medication and restraint, visits by the appointed Lunacy Commissioners, and a number of administration and financial records. These were also used by MacKenzie in her thesis on social factors in the admission, discharge and continuing stay of patients at Ticehurst (see MacKenzie, 1985, 1986).

TICEHURST HOUSE

Before describing the Casebooks themselves, it may be useful to give a brief account of Ticehurst House Asylum, which was founded in 1792 by Samuel Newington and run by successive members of the Newington family until 1917. It is still a private mental hospital using several of the nineteenth-century buildings. Set in some 300 acres of pleasant Sussex countryside, eight miles south-east of Tunbridge Wells, it became very much the most expensive and exclusive of private asylums during the nineteenth century. Fees were significantly greater than for any other private establishment and the provision of staff, rooms, facilities and recreations was lavish in the extreme. Thus, in 1845 the average cost of

patient care was three guineas per week, whereas fifteen shillings to two guineas was the average private asylum fee given in Parry-Jones's survey (Parry-Jones, 1972). By 1879, according to the thirty-third Annual Report of the Commissioners in Lunacy, Ticehurst cost some £470 p.a. By contrast, there were 72 private asylums that cost £200 p.a. or less, and 17 more costing £200–300 p.a. It is not surprising that during a meeting at Ticehurst of the south-eastern division of the Medico-Psychological Association (MPA) in October 1900 a Dr Bower should state that 'he had always looked forward to seeing Ticehurst, which he considered the Mecca of private asylums' (*Journal of Mental Science*, Jan. 1901, p. 73). At this same meeting the Newingtons outlined some of the features of the history and practices of their establishment (Medical Superintendents, 1901).

A central feature was 'the large staff employed', deemed to be 'a great blessing' by another visiting MPA member. In the 1850s there were some 100 attendants and servants of varying degrees, while by 1879 nearly 150 were employed. These were caring for some 60 patients between 1845 and 1865, and an average of 79 from 1875 to 1915. Additional villas were added to the licence during the latter part of the nineteenth century (Highlands, The Vineyards, Quarry Villa), buildings originally used as family residences by earlier generations of Newingtons. In 1864 houses were leased at St Leonards and in 1889 'we had a larger house specially built for us there'. These villas were managed by lady and gentleman superintendents who were expected to provide 'companionship' as well as 'domestic comfort', and each house was 'a social centre, between which invitations to tennis, cards, and tea are habitually exchanged'. By 1900 the Newingtons describe having six lady superintendents, and four gentlemen and four lady companions, the complement being made up by male attendants (75 % trained at Ticehurst) and female nurses, and a range of ordinary servants. The use of local families was widespread, and a number seem to have served at Ticehurst down and across the generations. The average length of service was 7·98 years in 1898 (10·04 for males, 5·5 for females), the higher turnover of females, who left to get married, being compensated for by their settling locally and providing a pool of experienced workers able to cover emergencies and holidays. Adopting the view that these attendants should behave as 'body servants or valets', the Newingtons relied on 'the exercise of common sense and the moral atmosphere' as the basis of treatment.

These human resources were aided by grounds and views ideal to John Conolly's (1847) notions. They were on 'a gentle eminence...and in a fertile and agreeable country, near enough to high roads...to facilitate the supply of stores, and the occasional visits of the friends of the patients, and to diversify the scene without occasioning disturbance'. Furthermore, Conolly wrote, 'if it is intended to receive patients of the educated classes into the house, it should unquestionably be situated amidst scenery calculated to give pleasure to such persons when of sane mind, those whose faculties have never been cultivated derive little satisfaction from the loveliest aspects of nature'. Such prescriptions were very much adhered to by the Newingtons, since carefully planned walks, arbours, summer houses and pleasure grounds were included on the site. There was a cricket pitch, a bowling lawn, a small golf course and even 'an aviary for gold and silver pheasants'. Some of these are depicted in an illustrated prospectus of 1830. Throughout the casenotes are constant references to walking, cricket and exercise, and it seems that some walking paths were specifically designed and measured so that certain distances could be prescribed for patients on an individual basis. In addition, since the 1820s there had been provided a pack of foot harriers to enable gentlemen to go hunting, since 'it ensures a large amount of physical exercise'. It is uncertain how successful this was since, 'unless a man has a special liking for the sport...it is most difficult to create any enthusiasm for it'. Finally, horses, carriages and dog-carts were widely used to ensure fresh air and external activity for those unable to exercise more vigorously, as recorded frequently in the notes and by other observers.

Indoor occupation was also lavish. Frequent lectures were provided (e.g. the Grossmiths visited on several occasions in the 1850s, and one patient made his escape during a lecture), while musical entertainments included 'weekly dances during the colder months' and performances by the establishment band twice a week. In fact, by the turn of the century all male attendants were expected to play an instrument. Tea parties, whist, private dinners and visits to the Newingtons were regular features, and it seems that the kudos of being invited to attend 'Miss Newington's table' was used to encourage good manners and propriety in those recovering from more disturbed states. Food and drink were plentiful, and concoctions of beef soup, porter and champagne were given to build up those refusing to eat or unable to feed properly. It does appear, however, that getting their rich clientele to partake actively in physical employment was difficult. 'We find it impossible to induce the class we have to deal with to undertake anything in the way of manual labour against their will', state the medical superintendents in 1901, and they went on to describe the expense incurred in laying out a large garden and greenhouse which had been rarely used, despite the gardening skills and interest of Dr Alexander Newington himself.

As for the Newington family, the details of their training and relationships are described in Mackenzie's work (1986). During 1845–90, the period of this study, three generations are prominent. Charles Newington (1781–1852), son of the founder, Samuel, ornamented the grounds and extended the asylum to his own house, Highlands. His sons, Charles (1813–1863) and Samuel (1814–1882), both qualified as physicians, via Cambridge and Oxford respectively, while their sons, Herbert Frances Hayes (1848–1917) and Alexander (1846–1914), both also trained in asylums (at Edinburgh and Bethlem) and took over the active running of Ticehurst from the late 1870s. Hayes ('H.H.N.' first writes clearly in the notes in September 1875) was certainly the most prominent, being President of the MPA in 1889–90 and Treasurer subsequently for many years (1894–1917) until his death. He wrote a number of articles for the *Journal of Mental Science*, was active in local politics and contributed practically to the development of training schemes for attendants and nurses. His obituarist (1917) asserted that 'to say that [he] was a many-sided man gives but a shadowy indication of the immensity of his activities and the diversity of his interests'. Described as 'the power not only "behind the throne" but by the side of successive presidents', as 'the most dominant personality at the Council' since the death of Hack Tuke and as 'a good cricketer, keen golfer and enthusiastic musician' (who 'did not think it derogatory to the dignity of his position to act as organist, choir-master and conductor of the orchestra of Ticehurst House'), he very much represents the spirit of the family and their methods of management during the last third of the nineteenth century. It is against this background that the Casebooks, their style and details, must be set.

THE CASEBOOKS

These provided the fundamental data for the study. Each one is clearly numbered and dated on the spine, and they seem to have been of a standard design to conform to the requirements of the 1845 Asylums Act ('An Act for the Regulation of the Case and Treatment of Lunatics'). Casebooks 1–32 cover the period 1846–90, when a new Lunacy Act was passed, partially changing the processes of admission to asylum care. In particular, voluntary patients became more prevalent.

Printed on the first two pages of each book are the rules of the Commissioners in Lunacy (whose signatures adorn the inside front cover) as to the procedure to be adopted in recording medical notes. Entitled 'Order as to the Case Book', this lays down stringent details concerning the information to be included, so that it may be 'easily referred to, and extracted, whenever the Commissioners shall so require'; they were amended in 1862.

Each book also contains an alphabetical index of the patients whose notes are contained therein, and is generally a mixture of detailed admission records for new patients and routine follow-up comments on those in for some time. One book may include admissions over several years, or simply for one year, but in general they proceed in a chronological fashion and it is not difficult to follow the course of an individual's admission from book to book. The end of one patient's notes is almost always marked with a reference to the volume and page number on which subsequent notes are to be found. Often an

admission note will occupy several sections in one book before being carried on two or three books later. Occasionally an admission will be chronologically aberrant, probably because empty pages in an old book were being filled in. Most books are full, varying in length from 150 to 350 pages, volumes 20–32 being especially thick.

The script is generally legible and in ink, with dates and names regularly stated for each entry. Handwriting varies over periods, the Newingtons initially recording the notes, but several assistant MOs (notably a Dr Francis Wilton from 1872 to 1882) predominate from the 1860s. Most notes are signed, and there is an increasing input of letters (e.g. those of William Gull, William Jenner, Henry Maudsley) from visiting physicians, as well as drawings, notes and letters written by the patients themselves. Details of medication are less easy to interpret because of the use of Latin shorthand for words and figures, but admission dates are very clear, as are the basic demographic data demanded by the Lunacy Commissioners.

The format of the notes alters over time, partly in response to the certification requirements, but more often because of the patient's condition or the author's degree of interest. Thus, the initial admission notes are often detailed and complex, but if a patient becomes chronic and unchanging the ritual of note-filling takes over. This leads to page after page of 'No change' or 'as usual' or 'in *status quo* mentally' or 'remains the same'. The official outcome of a case, whether by death or discharge, is also usually recorded, but there are notable omissions. Post-mortem examinations are few, but reported in full, as are causes of death. The official outcome terminology of 'recovered', 'relieved', 'not improved' can sometimes be obscured by the use of other terms (e.g. 'discharged', 'transferred to another asylum') and the Register of Discharges had to be used for clarification.

Because note-keeping was brought about only by the 1845 Act, the first Casebook is unique in recording a number of patients who had been in the asylum for many years, alongside new admissions between 1846 and 1850. It is very much a hotch-potch of variable detail. Thus a Mrs P. is described as dying on 11 March 1849, having been admitted on 13 May 1833. She was apparently married, but her age is not recorded. 'No improvement took place' and she died 'of old age'. Others are simply described as 'labouring under delusions for many years' or 'no change has taken place for many years'. On the other hand, there are entries covering 10–20 (or more) pages on several patients, such as Mr G. His personal details and past history are very full, as are the notes describing his mental state, behaviour and progress over the thirty-odd years from his admission in 1846 to his death, from pyaemia, in 1877. These are not of course all contained in Casebook 1, but they do illustrate the gradual evolution of the notes from the brief comments of 1846 to the elaborate details that pertain from 1851. For it is from this date that the standard outline emerges, in which a detailed physical examination, previous personal and medical history, family history and mental state are routinely recorded. Mrs Elwes, admitted on 17 February 1851, is the first recipient of this kind of detail (see below for further details of the case). By the 1860s the contents of the medical certificates are increasingly being recorded verbatim in the notes, although much of the 'previous history' was probably derived from these anyway prior to this date. Likewise, formal descriptions of 'temperament' and head shape are included more and more in the physical examination (e.g. 'highly nervous' or 'melancholic' temperament; head 'well formed' or 'natural'), while the 'present (mental) state' becomes more elaborate. By the mid-1870s a standardized description of new admissions is emerging, wherein the cause, course, and circumstances are routinely appended, along with 'Yes/No' comments as to the presence of epilepsy, dangerousness and suicidal tendencies. Examples of casenotes, edited by the author, are in the appendix (see pp. 64–67).

The continuation notes also follow a standard format, being written daily, then weekly, then monthly, and only resorting to a three-monthly (four times a year) comment when the patient was deemed incurable. In general notes written after a month or so are routine, concentrating on behaviour, minor physical concerns and medication. Thus, Mrs O. (p. 264, Vol. 26) is described on 15 May 1881, some two months after her fourth admission, as suffering 'from a little debility – attends the parish church and

chapel in the house. Her conversation is rational and she seems to realise that her mind has been affected'. Unfortunately, her relapse into violence is such that she later has to be transferred elsewhere (she 'smashed a marble mantelpiece' and 'threw a stone at H.H.N.'), but this description at least gives an indication of social interaction that assists in differentiating between chronic and relapsing states. However, it is not uncommon for patients, long hiding behind the obscurity of routine notes, to emerge in a new light when a more detailed comment is appended. Overall, therefore, the Casebooks are never entirely static, changes in language and detail constantly refreshing the picture of individual patients. They certainly provide a 'discourse of practice' (Ray, 1981) untainted by any expectation of publication or social effect.

ASSESSMENT PROCEDURE

Given these documents from this asylum, it was necessary to formulate a means of obtaining information that would be useful, coherent and objective in the process of diagnosis. The first task was to ensure that the data were sufficiently detailed for the kinds of analysis proposed. Since Casebook 1 was so variable (see above), Casebooks 2 and 3 were studied as well, using the International Classification of Diseases (ICD-9) Glossary (1978) as a reference for diagnoses. In general, it seemed clear that a majority of cases post-1850 fitted the diagnostic outlines of ICD-9. Six cases were therefore extracted and edited and sent to eight psychiatrists for their diagnostic assessment before a routine research meeting. At this meeting the problem of attempting retrospective diagnosis was discussed and opinions sought on the six cases. For the first five cases the degree of unanimity was exceptional, all present agreeing independently about the most likely diagnosis with the exception of one participant, who disagreed on one of the cases but agreed on the other four. The sixth case could find no consensus and the author's opinion of 'unknown' for the diagnosis was confirmed. There was, however, agreement as to there being insufficient grounds for coming to a definite decision.

With such confirmation as to the reliability of the diagnostic procedure, the Casebooks were systematically examined up to the end of Volume

32 – in all approximately 8000 pages of written notes. Each case was numbered and recorded in two separate ways. The name and number, with age, sex, marital status and discharge dates were recorded both on a card and on a separate foolscap sheet of paper. On the card was also recorded outcome (if apparent) and likely diagnosis according to ICD-9 criteria, which are verbal descriptions, and Research Diagnostic Criteria (RDC) as developed for DSM-III. Notes as to whether violence (V), restraint (R), alcohol abuse (ETOH), movement disorder (M) or particular symptoms were reported were also made, as was a computation of the length of stay in years and months. These basic data were recorded additionally on the more detailed foolscap sheets, along with descriptions of the mental and physical state, behavioural and psychological changes reported in the notes and social data. In effect, this second set of records was a précis of the Casebook notes, and descriptions of relevant psychopathology were transcribed in full when of especial interest. The collation of this information went on in parallel, working chronologically through the Case-books. At one point four admissions were left out, and this accounts for several minor anomalies in the enumeration of the cases in the results.

Once this primary task was finished a third database was established, recording the cases in alphabetical order on a second set of cards. This involved going through the case summaries and record cards again, reassessing diagnostic decisions, and making specific notes on a number of phenomena that were well recorded originally. Simultaneously, the Admission and Discharge Registers were studied to cross-check the Case-book data and supplement it where necessary. In particular, the diagnosis used at the time of admission was recorded, along with the data on symptoms and treatments so as to provide a full picture of correlations for subsequent analysis in the light of the modern diagnosis.

Specific information was obtained in the following areas.

(A) Delusions

All descriptions of delusional beliefs were recorded in brief according to diagnosis and patient's number. The use of the word 'delusions' above was not sufficient. To be included in this category a clear record of the nature of the patient's abnormal belief was necessary. Thus a Mr T. (No. 136) claimed a 'bug has crawled into his ear', Miss M. (No. 240) said she was 'the Virgin Mary' and Mr F. (No. 579) insisted he had 'no legs or mouth'.

(B) Hallucinations

As with delusions, descriptions of patients' acting under the influence of, or personally recounting, hallucinatory experiences were included here. The phrases 'auditory' or 'aural hallucinations' are not used until 1877, although the register of admissions records 'Hallucinations of Hearing, etc.' as one diagnosis in 1866 and 'hysterical Mania with Hallucinations' in 1867. The terms 'voice(s)' and 'visions' are used with increasing frequency, as with Mr D. (No. 334), who 'knows his wife is in India, but hears her voice constantly talking to him' (1874), or Mr T. (No. 350), who 'hears conversations through the floor or through the wainscot' (1875). To qualify for inclusion under this heading the psychopathological description had to be repeated at least twice and to describe a behaviour associated with 'hearing voices', etc.

(C) Movement/posture disorder

In view of modern concern as to the bases of tardive dyskinesia and catatonic symptoms, a cohort of patients untouched by modern pharmacotherapy should provide useful data as to the natural prevalence of such conditions. All patients were therefore additionally screened for descriptions of persistent or recurrent abnormalities of movement and/or posture. Given the concentration on behaviour, as opposed to psychology, in these notes, this search was most rewarding. Patients described simply as 'restless' or 'agitated' were so frequent that this term was not deemed sufficient for inclusion in this category. More specific phrases as 'ugly grimaces', 'constant fidgetting' or 'adopts all sorts of positions' and 'extraordinary attitudes' were required, repeated on more than one or two occasions. As with the category 'Masturbation', the data were correlated with age, sex, marital status, length of stay, modern diagnosis and, in addition, outcome.

(D) Masturbation

The frequent references to self-abuse and masturbation were recorded in view of the aetiological significance attributed to this behaviour during the latter part of the nineteenth century (Hare, 1962), in particular after David Skae's theories became prominent. Data on age, sex, marital status, modern diagnosis, length of stay and associated disorders were collected for those patients described more than once as 'masturbating' or 'abusing themselves'.

(E) Specific psychopathology

(i) *Flight of ideas*

Examples of this symptom were collected since it has a particular relationship to the thought/language disorder of a manic illness. It is also a specific symptom in the RDC contributing to the diagnosis of 'mania' or 'hypomania'. The phrase was not used in itself by the physicians at Ticehurst, so only transcriptions of patients' statements that fitted this symptom were used. Thus, Mr B. (No. 221) 'soon loses the thread and goes to another subject', while Mrs P. 'flies from one subject to another'.

(ii) *Passivity experience*, (iii) *Negative symptoms*, (iv) *Thought disorder*

Clear descriptions of these symptoms were collected, in order to correlate them with the diagnoses and disorders outlined above. This was to illustrate the 'stability of psychopathological phenomena in a shifting psychosocial matrix of description', to quote Berrios (1985, personal communication). The Appendix contains detailed examples of individual cases and symptom profiles.

(F) Unusual disorders

An attempt was made to take especial note of symptoms and signs associated with the less-common neurological and psychiatric disorders such as (i) Capgras syndrome, (ii) Cotard's syndrome (nihilistic delusion), (iii) eating disorders (bulimia and anorexia nervosa), (iv) neurological syndromes (e.g. Korsakoff's psychosis), (v) non-psychotic disorders (e.g. phobic disorder), (vi) puerperal illness, (vii) erotomania. This was in part to look for evidence of 'stability of psychological phenomena' (see 'E' above), in part to enhance the picture of the disorders presenting in the nineteenth century.

(G) Treatment approaches

(i) *Drugs*

The widespread use of various drugs, including bromide, chloral, *Cannabis indica* (Indian hemp), etc., was apparent, although the details could not be systematically recorded without a better understanding of shorthand prescriptions. However, the dates of certain drugs first being used were noted, and the requirement for stomach pumps, mustard baths and electrical treatments (e.g. 'galvanization' or 'faradization') was fully detailed. The prevalence of such physical treatments could thus be computed, along with the symptoms and diagnoses for which they were applied.

(ii) *Numerical data*

The use of numerical, as opposed to descriptive, accounts of patients' status was recorded, so as to illustrate changes in the various assessment procedures.

(iii) *Cricket*

The use of cricket as an occupation, form of exercise or even therapy seems to have been a particular activity of the asylum. Some details of those patients partaking in this game are appended, largely to illustrate the background *zeitgeist* of the place and the role of organized sport as a means of assessing both abnormality of behaviour and response to treatment.

(H) Violence/restraint

In view of the prevalence of such behaviour, and the increasingly rare use of overt restraint (i.e. mechanical devices such as the camisole), details of these behaviours were collected and related to age, sex and diagnosis. Such data seemed particularly pertinent in terms of assessing the role of the asylum and its attendants in coping with difficult behaviours.

(I) Alcohol

The prevalence of alcohol abuse, as a significant factor prior to admission, was recorded and related to age, sex and diagnosis. In view of the varying sources of personal histories, it is doubtful whether these data were especially reliable. For example, no mention of alcohol is made in the history of a physician admitted in a state of clear 'delirium tremens'.

(J) Suicide

Only three patients committed suicide while under care at Ticehurst. One other death may have been deliberately induced. Details were recorded.

The perusal of the Casebooks was thus undertaken with particular reference to those topics listed, their prevalence being checked during the subsequent reanalysis of the primary data.

Alongside this process went that of making diagnoses. As stated above, this used the ICD-9 and the RDC. Such operational criteria have no especial historic validity (Kendell, 1989) but are reliable in ensuring coherence of diagnosis across individuals and cultures, and are now widely used in research studies. Their usage implies an hierarchical view of diagnosis, as described by Foulds (1976), in that the presence of clear organic pathology takes precedence over psychological phenomena, and psychotic illness overrides neurosis. They were generally easy to apply to the available notes, because details of sleep, appetite, behaviour, and social interaction were so well recorded that the less obvious descriptions of psychological symptoms were sometimes unnecessary for a diagnosis to be reached. The categories used by the RDC are complex, but for the purposes of this study subgroups were rarely used. In essence the diagnoses could be divided into five main groups as follows.

(i) *'Schizophrenias'*

Probable or definite, including 'catatonic', 'acute' and schizoaffective disorders, although the latter were recorded as well.

(ii) *'Manic-depressive disorders'*

Probable or definite, which included major depressive disorder, mania and bipolar illnesses.

(iii) *'Organic illnesses'*

These were given a high priority and attributed with a low threshold of suspicion. The evidence of a concurrent physical illness (e.g. uraemia) normally meant that an 'organic' diagnosis was made. The major problem was the role of 'General paralysis of the insane' (GPI), since a number of patients came in with purely psychological symptoms (e.g. mania) before developing physical signs. On the second analysis a number of diagnoses were changed to 'organic' (GPI) because of this. Likewise alcohol-withdrawal came under this category even if outstanding affective or schizophreniform symptoms were apparent.

(iv) *'Neurotic disorders'*

Primarily this group contained the 'minor depressive disorder' category of the RDC and was used to categorize patients who lacked the symptoms to be included in group (ii). Several obsessional and phobic illnesses are also found here.

(v) *'Indefinite'* (*'?'*)

When no clear diagnosis could be reached, this was used, in particular during the early part of the study when notes were very sparse. All patients 'began' with this as their description, and the subsequent attribution of a diagnosis therefore had to be a positive step of accumulating suitable data.

Results

The overall diagnostic picture of Ticehurst Asylum patients can be seen in Table 1. Using the five broad categories of 'schizophrenia' (S); 'manic-depressive disorder' (MD); 'organic illness' (O); 'neurotic illness' (N) and 'indefinite' (?), these results have been organized into quinquennia between 1845 and 1889, with the pre-1845 and post-1889 data appended. While there is variation across individual years, particularly in the number of admissions (averaging 5 p.a. in the early 1850s to 19 p.a. in the early 1880s) the annual spread of diagnoses generally conforms to the quinquennial pattern. The lowest number of admissions recorded in a single year is three, occurring in 1847, 1852 (the year of a fire in the main building) and 1858. The highest number is 24, in 1883 and 1884.

Of those deemed 'schizophrenic', 56 are 'probable' and 101 'definite' instances of that diagnosis. In addition, 16 fulfil the DSM-III criteria for schizoaffective disorder, but I have subsumed this diagnosis under the category of 'schizophrenia' in view of its nosological uncertainty and as an aid to simplifying the range of diagnoses.

It will be noted that the proportion of 'indefinite' diagnoses is especially high in the pre-1845 and 1845–9 cohorts (75% and 50% respectively), whereas the 'manic-depressive' group is non-existent. If these early patients are eliminated from the analysis, the total percentage of such diagnoses is considerably altered, the 'manic-depressive' group increasing to 215/515, namely 41·7%, while the 'indefinites' fall to 54/515, which is 10·5%. Other categories are only minimally affected. Since nearly half (53/107) of those deemed 'indefinite' come into the early, poorly documented phase of the Casebooks, these adjusted figures will be given due weight in the Discussion.

In overall terms, the proportion of 'schizophrenia' admissions is consistently about a quarter (26%) of the total, with the exception of the 1850–4 cohort. With the same exception the proportion of 'manic-depressives' is regularly between one-third and one-half of the total, while the 'indefinite' and 'neurotic' figures occupy some 10% and 5% respectively. Most variation is seen in the 'organic' category, embracing a range of physical illness, mainly

Table 1. *Modern diagnosis of Ticehurst patients, 1845–1890*

| Admission date | Total admissions | Diagnosis (% per quinquennium)* | | | | |
		Schizophrenic	Manic-depressive	Organic	Neurotic	Indefinite
Pre-1845	52	11 (21)	—	2 (4)	—	39 (75)
1845–9	28	4 (14)	—	5 (18)	5 (18)	14 (50)
1850–4	25	12 (48)	6 (24)	2 (8)	1 (4)	4 (16)
1855–9	22	6 (28)	11 (50)	2 (9)	2 (9)	1 (4)
1860–4	58	19 (33)	22 (38)	7 (12)	3 (5)	7 (12)
1865–9	84	20 (24)	31 (37)	21 (25)	2 (2)	10 (12)
1870–4	69	22 (32)	24 (35)	11 (16)	4 (6)	8 (11)
1875–9	90	21 (23)	47 (52)	9 (10)	6 (7)	7 (8)
1880–4	96	16 (17)	46 (48)	19 (20)	7 (7)	8 (8)
1885–9	71	26 (37)	28 (39)	7 (10)	1 (1)	9 (13)
Totals	595	157 (26)	215 (36)	85 (15)	31 (5)	107 (18)
1890	2	—	1	—	—	1
1893–1916	4	1	1	1	—	1
Overall	601	158	217	86	31	109

* Percentages to nearest whole number.

Table 2. *Diagnostic terms, from admission registers, for patients fulfilling modern diagnosis of 'schizophrenia', 1850–1889, by decennia*

Contemporary diagnosis or phrase	1850–9 (%)	1860–9 (%)	1870–9 (%)	1880–9 (%)	Total usage (%)
Delusions	15 (83·5)	16 (41)	27 (62·8)	11 (26·2)	69 (48·6)
(Delusions + phrase)	(5)	(4)	(24)	(7)	—
Dementia	1 (5·5)	2 (5)	1 (2·3)	2 (4·8)	6 (4·2)
Auditory/aural hallucinations*	—	[3] 1 (2·5)	[3] —	[1] 7 (16·7)	8 (5·6)
Mania (±phrase)†	—	8 (20·5)	7 (16·3)	16 (38·0)	31 (21·8)
Melancholia	—	—	2 (4·7)	3 (7·1)	5 (3·5)
Monomania	—	3 (8)	—	—	3 (2·1)
Imbecility/mental enfeeblement	—	2 (5)	1 (2·3)	1 (2·4)	4 (2·9)
Chorea	1 (5·5)	—	—	—	1 (0·8)
Descriptive phrases	1 (5·5)	—	5 (11·6)	—	6 (4·2)
Nil used	—	7 (18)	—	2 (4·8)	9 (6·3)
Totals	18	39	43	42	142

* Figures in square brackets indicate that the term 'hallucinations' has been used additionally in a phrase subordinate to 'delusions'.
† The term 'mania' has also been used subordinate to 'delusions' as part of the 'delusions + phrase' group. This occurs 7 times in 1870–9 and 4 times in 1880–9.

GPI (this provides 10 of the 21 cases between 1865 and 1869), alcohol-induced syndromes and epilepsy.

Tables 2–4 describe the contemporary diagnostic terms used for three of the modern categories over the 1850–89 period. Other notable terms used include the phrase 'delusional insanity' (which has been recorded here in the 'delusions' category), 'suicidal' or 'suicidal tendency' (usually part of the 'delusions + phrase' category), and 'religious', to describe both delusions and monomania. The 'descriptive phrases', that are particularly common in the 1870s, include such terms as 'excitement', 'confusion', 'influence of imaginary voices' and 'addressed imaginary persons... seldom gives a rational answer' (see Table 2). The term 'monomania' was additionally used once in the notes of an 1850s case but has not been included here.

The most striking feature is the decline in the use of the term 'delusions' (from over three-quarters to just over one-quarter of the diagnoses used), the increasing diversity of language, and increased use of the phrase 'chronic mania'.

The 'descriptive phrases' used include 'capable of answering' and terms like 'unsound... insane... mind feeble' (see Table 3). Again, the increasing diversity of language is noteworthy, as is the switch from 'delusions' to forms of 'mania'. The proportion deemed 'mania' during the 1880s (7/17, which is 41·2%) is very similar to the 1880s 'schizophrenia' group (38%) (see Table 2).

Table 3. *Diagnostic terms, from admission registers, of patients categorized as 'indefinite' ('?'), 1850–1889, by decennia*

Contemporary phrase or diagnosis	1850–9	1860–9	1870–9	1880–9	Total usage (%)
Delusions	*3 (2)	4	1	2	10 (18·5)
Dementia	—	3	1	3	7 (12·9)
Mania	1	2†	6†	7†	16 (29·6)
Melancholia	—	—	2	2	4 (7·4)
Monomania	—	1	—	—	
Imbecile	1	—	—	—	
General paralysis‡	—	1	—	—	
Nymphomania	—	1	—	—	11 (20·5)
Moral insanity	—	—	—	2	
Senile insanity	—	—	—	1	
Descriptive phrases	—	—	4	—	
Nil used	—	5	1	—	6 (11·1)
Decennial totals	5	17	15	17	54

* In two instances a phrase is attached, as 'subject to paroxysms of excitement'.
† In the 1860s this is 'hysterical mania' and in the 1870s four cases are prefixed 'chronic'.
‡ This is the first, and isolated, use of the phrase 'General paralysis', used once more in 1868 and 1867, then neglected until the 1880s (at least as an *initial* diagnosis).

The trends noted in Tables 2 and 3 continue in Table 4, in that 'mania' becomes markedly more popular; by the 1880s 'mania' and 'melancholia' comprise over 80% of the diagnoses, while these two terms and 'delusions'

Table 4. *Diagnostic terms, from admission registers, for patients fulfilling criteria for 'manic-depressive disorder', 1850–1889, by decennia*

Contemporary diagnosis or phrase	1850–9 (%)	1860–9 (%)	1870–9 (%)	1880–9 (%)	Total usage (%)
Delusions (delusions	11 (64·7)	19 (35·8)	23 (32·4)	7 (9·4)	60 (27·8)
+ phrase)	(4)	(5)	(20)	(7)	
Dementia	—	2 (3·8)	—	—	2 (1·0)
Mania*	4 (23·5)	13 (24·5)	21 (29·6)	33 (44·4)	71 (33·0)
Melancholia†	2 (11·8)	6 (11·3)	18 (25·3)	27 (36·4)	53 (24·6)
Erotomania	—	1 (1·9)	—	—	1 (0·5)
Senile insanity/dementia	—	—	1 (1·4)	1 (1·4)	2 (1·0)
Depression	—	—	—	1 (1·4)	1 (0·5)
Moral insanity	—	—	—	1 (1·4)	1 (0·5)
Hysterical insanity	—	—	—	1 (1·4)	1 (0·5)
General paralysis?	—	—	—	1 (1·4)	1 (0·5)
Descriptive phrase/term‡	—	1 (1·9)	8 (11·3)	1 (1·4)	10 (4·6)
Nil used	—	11 (20·8)	—	1 (1·4)	12 (5·5)
Totals	17	53	71	74	215

* The term 'mania' is usually prefixed with 'acute' or 'subacute', but 'hysterical', 'senile', 'puerperal', 'recurrent', 'paroxysmal', 'suicidal' and 'violent' are also used, as is 'chronic' twice. It also often has an attached phrase or term, and is subordinated to 'delusions'.
† This term is used in phrases with 'delusions' and sometimes with 'mania', but has been subordinated in this analysis.
‡ These include 'unsocial ... kicks out', 'suicidal ... refuses food', 'nervous ... hesitating' and 'weak manner ... peculiar', as well as the term 'hypochondriasis'.

comprise over 85% of the diagnostic terms overall. This homogeneity contrasts clearly with the greater diversity noted elsewhere. The phrase 'aural hallucinations' is recorded only once, secondary to 'acute mania' in 1879.

It should be noted how the term 'delusions' is increasingly given a descriptive phrase, used on its own seven times (out of 11) in the 1850s, three times (out of 23) in the 1870s and never in the 1880s, when it goes into decline.

The 'nil used' section (i.e. no diagnosis has been written down) follows the trend of Tables 2 and 3 also, in that the 1860s are overrepresented here (11 times).

It is of interest to note the similar diagnostic language of the Admissions Register between 1890 and 1906. Of 171 entries traced, 60 (35·1%) were termed 'mania' (with or without a prefix, such as 'acute', or an accompanying phrase), 41 were termed 'melancholia', 19 'dementia', 10 'general paralysis' and 14 were given no diagnosis. Of the remainder only 10 were termed 'delusional insanity', three 'moral insanity' and two 'depression'. Other phrases included 'insanity of adolescence' (on a 23-year-old male in 1893, caused apparently by anaemia of the brain), 'insanity of negations' ('he says he does not exist, that he died some years ago'), 'insanity of persecution' (twice), and 'insanity of con-

duct', but these novel diagnoses are still very much the exception.

The cohort was also divided, according to length of stay, into three groups for analysis by modern diagnosis, outcome as recorded in the Casebooks and registers, age, sex, and marital status. The three groups consisted of:
(a) those admitted for 1 year or less, numbering 280;
(b) those admitted for 1–5 years, numbering 127;
(c) those admitted for 5 years or longer, numbering 105.

Discharge date was by certificate, which normally coincided with leaving the asylum, although some patients actually went out earlier on leave/trial, while others stayed on as voluntary boarders, or in the vicinity with an attendant or nurse. Those admitted prior to 1850 (80 patients) and a number of others whose discharge date was unclear were excluded.

The average age for the whole cohort was 42·72 years, although prior to 1865 it was 38·70 and between 1866 and 1875 it was 46·36, before settling to the average.

A summary of the data for all three 'length of stay' groupings is shown in Table 5. As can be seen from this table, increasing length of stay is associated with a younger age on admission,

Table 5. *Length of stay of Ticehurst patients (1850–1889) by age, sex, marital status, modern diagnosis and outcome*

	< 1 year	1–5 years	> 5 years
Total nos.	280	127	105
Average age	45·53	45·05	41·76
Male/female ratio (%)	132/148 (0·89)	78/49 (1·59)	54/51 (1·06)
Single/married ratio (%)	134/146 (0·92)	71/56 (1·27)	72(1)/32 (2·25)
	Diagnosis (%)		
Schizophrenic	(17·5)	(22·0)	(60·0)
Manic-depressive	(52·9)	(38·6)	(16·2)
Organic	(15·0)	(24·4)	(8·6)
Neurotic	(7·1)	(4·7)	—
Indefinite	(7·5)	(10·3)	(15·2)
	Outcome (%)		
Died	(12·1)	(32·0)	(82·8)
Recovered/cured	(53·6)	(20·3)	(1·0)
Relieved	(15·4)	(21·9)	(5·7)
Not improved, etc.	(18·9)	(25·8)	(10·5)

single status, a diagnosis of 'schizophrenia' or 'indefinite' and an insignificant rate of recovery or even relief.

A stay of less than 1 year is associated with being older, married, 'manic-depressive' or 'neurotic' and a relatively good outcome, more than half being 'recovered' or 'relieved'.

The medium stay of 1–5 years is particularly associated with organic illness and being male, which may reflect the impact of GPI.

MOVEMENT AND POSTURE

A total of 73 patients were clearly identified as having a significant disorder of movement or posture not due to an identifiable physical deformity or neurological illness. Of these, 45 were 'schizophrenic' and 24 had an 'indefinite' diagnosis. One of the remaining four was a 52-year-old widow admitted for three months in 1876 with 'acute mania'. She was described as having 'actions rapid and jerky ... her hands and head are not still for a second', among a host of other symptoms such as 'restlessness' and 'chattering incoherence' with 'a tendency to hilarious excitement'. She recovered fully and had several relapses subsequently but never again were the 'jerky' movements described. The remaining three had organic illness. A 44-year-old physician was 'touching everything with one finger', ritualistically, while uraemic; a

72-year-old diplomat was 'constantly making faces', and a 36-year-old guards colonel had a 'constant grinding movement' of his jaw. Both the latter had other symptoms of probable (but unconfirmed) GPI.

Additional phenomena noted in this group included thought disorder (11), passivity experiences (8) and violent behaviour (30), five of whom required restraint. Ten patients fitted the definitions of catatonia in the RDC, and one (a 56-year-old single woman) 'seldom opens her mouth except to utter involuntary bad names' while persistently 'fidgetting', striking and pinching people. Being also described as 'of dwarfish stature', with a 'flat face' and 'imbecile expression', and 'having a crop of molluscum' on her face, it may be she had Tourette's syndrome associated with a degree of mental retardation.

The cohort was also noteworthy for being predominantly single (55 out of 73), and male (42 out of 73).

Overall, some 28% of the Ticehurst schizophrenics and 22% of the 'indefinites' come into this category (see Table 6), which seems to indicate not only a relationship between the two categories but a very high proportion of movement/posture disorder. Outcome is poor (only 14/73, or 19·1%, are ever 'recovered/relieved') and chronicity is marked.

MASTURBATION

The first use of this term in the Ticehurst material was in 1862 when masturbation was 'the supposed cause of the attack' in a 26-year-old gentleman. The terms 'self-abuse' and 'abusing himself/herself' then increasingly came into use as well. Altogether, 70 patients were described as indulging in this behaviour. Since patient No. 150 in my records was the first, potentially at least 451 more could have been included, giving an overall (though parsimonious) incidence of 15·5%. It is likely to have been considerably higher.

The characteristics of this group were analysed. There was a small predominance of males (41 out of 70 (58·6%)), 27 (38·6%) additionally evinced a disorder of movement/posture, 35 (50%) were violent and the commonest diagnostic category was 'schizophrenia' (40 out of 70 (57·1%)). A further 16 were 'manic-de-

Table 6. *Modern diagnoses of Ticehurst House patients, 1845–1890, relating them to length of stay, outcome, sex, mental status, movement/posture disorder, violence and masturbation (percentages)*

	Schizophrenia	Manic-depressive	Organic	Neurotic	Indefinite
Total (%)	26	36	15	5	18
Length of stay					
< 1 year	35	69	51	77	42
1–5 years	20	23	38	23	26
> 5 years	45	8	11	—	32
Overall outcome					
Died*	38·6	16·8	59·8	7·7	40
Cured/recovered	18·6	52·8	21·9	42·3	18
Relieved	10·7	17·3	7·3	46·2	14
Discharged/not improved	32·1	13·1	11·0	3·8	28
Gender					
Male	50·7	40·7	84·1	42·3	48
Female	49·3	59·3	15·9	57·7	52
Marital status					
Single	71·4†	42·5	45·1	30·8	80
Married	27·9	57·5	54·9	69·2	20
Having a movement or posture disorder	28·5	0·5	3·6	—	22
Described as masturbating	28·6	7·5	4·9	—	20
Described as violent	35·7	23·8	15·9	—	40

* Includes patients who stayed in asylum for rest of life.   † One schizophrenic has no clear marital status.

pressive' (22·9%), 10 were 'indefinite' (14·3%) and four had organic disorders (5·7%), three of which were GPI. The increasing use of the term is particularly apparent in the 1880s for both new and chronic patients.

This language of masturbation not only increases in frequency, but also in its mode of usage. From being merely a description of behaviour, sometimes given nosological significance, it is used more and more as a cause of behaviour. Thus, Mr B's (No. 203) 'self-abuse continues' in 1876 and he has become 'restless and noisy owing to his bad habit of masturbating' in 1889. Similarly Mr J. (No. 253) is admitted in 1869, 'abuses himself' – alongside 'talks to the voices', 'absurd costumes', 'scribbling notes', etc. – in 1876, while in 1884 he is 'complaining of dyspepsia' or 'very irritable', ... 'probably owing to his masturbatory practices'.

VIOLENCE

The total number of those deemed violent, and described as such, was 134, 64 being male. This is 22·3% of the whole cohort of 601, and given the limited information on the pre-1851 admissions may well be an underestimate. Fifty (37·3%) had a diagnosis of 'schizophrenia', 51 (38·1%)

were 'manic-depressive', 20 (14·9%) were 'indefinite' and 13 (9·7%) had organic disorders, 10 of these being GPI. The average age on admission was 36·81 years, markedly younger than the 42·72 years of the whole cohort.

Restraint was used, according to the Casebooks, in only 28 patients (including one patient twice during separate admissions), 25 instances being before 1870.

In order to demonstrate the overall relationship between diagnosis, length of stay, outcome, sex, marital status, movement disorder, masturbation and violence, Table 6 was constructed using percentage figures. This provides a composite statistical picture of the demography and behaviours of the major diagnostic groups.

Outlines of the treatment approaches used per decennium are shown in Table 7, comparing them with total admissions and the incidence of violence for the same periods. The proportion of violent patients, overall 27·5%, varies from 29·8% in the 1850s to 20·8% in the 1870s. By contrast, restraint is used in 35·7% of violent cases in the 1850s and 32·5% in the 1860s, but drops to 3% and 4·8% in the 1870s and 1880s.

Tables 8A and 8B show summaries of a randomly selected cohort of 100 consecutive

Table 7. *Treatment approaches (restraint, mustard baths, stomach pump, electricity) and incidence of violence at Ticehurst from pre-1849 to 1889, compared to total admissions*

	Total	Recorded violence	Restraint	Mustard baths	Stomach pump	Electricity
Pre-1849	80	5	7*	—	—	—
1850–9	47	14	5	—	3	—
1860–9	142	40	13	10	14	2
1870–9	159	33	1	18	23	1
1880–9	167	42	2	10	14	7
Totals	595	134	28	38	54	10
% of total admissions		22·5	4·7	6·4	9·0	1·7

* The greater figures for restraint than violence is clearly anomalous, reflecting the inadequate details of the notes and several long-stay patients admitted pre-1849 but not recorded as under restraint until much later.

Table 8 (a). *Outcome of patients admitted to Ticehurst House, deemed at risk of suicide, from 100 consecutive admissions (January 1876 to June 1881) by RDC diagnosis*

Diagnosis	Average age (years)	Died	Not improved	Improved/ relieved	Recovered/ cured	Total
Schizophrenia	34·8	1*	3	1	0	5
Manic-depressive†	46·7	1*	2	9	4	16
Organic	29·0	1	0	0	0	1
Neurotic‡	45·8	1	1	3	2	7
Indefinite	31·0	0	0	2	0	2
Totals		4	6	15	6	31

* Committed suicide.
† Only one of the manic-depressive patients was in a manic phase (she had recovered).
‡ All neurotics fulfilled 'minor depression' criteria on the RDC.
N.B.: 15 were male, 16 female and 5 exhibited violent behaviour at some time during admission.

Table 8 (b). *Outcome of patients admitted to Ticehurst House, deemed at risk of suicide from 100 consecutive admissions (January 1876 to June 1881) by contemporary diagnosis*

Diagnosis	Died	Not improved	Improved/ relieved	Recovered/ cured	Total
Melancholia	2*	3	10	5	20
Mania, etc.	2*	1	3	1	7
Other terms	—	2	2	—	4
Totals	4	6	15	6	31

* One melancholic and one patient diagnosed 'chronic mania' committed suicide.

admissions about whom the characteristics of those deemed at risk of suicide have been extracted. At least 31 patients were thus classified, usually fulfilling 'manic-depressive' or 'neurotic' criteria in modern terms (22 out of 31) or 'melancholia' (20 out of 31) in contemporary terms. The positive outcome ('relieved/improved/recovered/cured') in 21 cases (67%) is a contrast to other selected groups.

Discussion

This array of numerical and descriptive results has been focused on collating clinical data so as to clarify diagnosis and management in a Victorian asylum. The reliability and validity of these findings will be discussed, with regard to both the diagnostic process and the representative nature of the cohort as a whole. Certain areas of clinical concern, such as the evidence for movement disorder akin to tardive dyskinesia, the symptoms seen as indicating mental illness, and the treatments for specific conditions, will be analysed in some depth. Extending the significance of this material into the wider debate, as to the ethos and role of nineteenth-century asylums, is limited by the fine focus of the study. Six hundred patients, in an exclusive private establishment, may be seen as too socially selected for useful comparisons. Nevertheless, there do seem to be some important general points relevant to present historical concerns and uncertainties.

Some broad conclusions should perhaps be initially outlined, because they have emerged directly from the business of working through the Casebook material. The most striking of these is the recognizability of the cases recorded. In over 80 % it has been possible to reach a form of broad diagnosis as judged by modern criteria. Even in those cases described as 'uncertain' there has rarely been behaviour or courses of illness that seem strange or clinically novel. Given the previous attempts at diagnosing such case records (Klaf & Hamilton, 1961: James & May 1981), this may not seem surprising to clinical psychiatrists, but such attempts were confined to schizophrenic symptoms, using non-operational criteria (Klaf & Hamilton, 1961), or to textbook cases of Kraepelin's dementia praecox (James & May, 1981). This thesis extends and reinforces such approaches, showing the consistency of certain symptom patterns over the last 140 years. Foucault's extended notion (1967) that 'we are not dealing with the same madmen' finds no support. Certain phrases, behaviours, and reactions were extraordinarily redolent of modern clinical psychiatry, whether in terms of positive symptoms such as flight of ideas or thought insertion, or chronic, negative habits such as 'lying on the sofa' or 'excessively fond of tobacco'. Such recognizability was of course central to any further analysis using a clinical perspective.

Associated with this was the severity of symptoms portrayed. By contrast to modern practice, the florid psychotic material and disturbed patterns of behaviour were striking. Depressive and manic states were often characterized by delusions and hallucinations concerning 'unpardonable sins' or reinforcing grandiose ideas. Chronic psychotic illness, usually schizophrenic, was accompanied by violence, incontinence of urine and faeces, unpleasant eating habits and overt masturbation. Such behaviours are well recognized by modern clinicians but their accumulation and persistence in one establishment is becoming a thing of the past. Writing of his own experiences in an asylum in 1929, Parfitt (1985) described admissions as 'far gone, roughly the worst fifth of modern admissions, neglected until psychosis, with bizarre delusions and riotous hallucinations, patently intolerable in the community'. The Ticehurst material very much reflects this kind of experience, and Victorian methods of management must be judged in the light of such phenomena. To what extent this severity is a special case, representing the 'worst fifth' of wealthy lunatics brought into an asylum as a last desperate measure, is clearly a subject for debate. Given the number of patients 'removed' for bad behaviour, and the material elegance and style of Ticehurst House itself, there are good grounds for suggesting that the clientele was not untypical of the times, or even biased towards a more amenable category.

Of course one factor influencing clinical presentations may well have been physical illness. At least 86 (15%) of the cases had 'organic' diagnoses, particularly general paralysis of the insane (GPI), which comprised nearly half of this group (48%). Another 20% were alcohol-related conditions, with epilepsy, other forms of brain damage, and occasional metabolic or febrile disorders making up the numbers. Given the similarity of symptoms between manic-depressive illness and the early stages of GPI, it is likely that a number of patients discharged 'relieved' or 'recovered' from apparent affective disorders would have gone on to develop overt paralytic illness. Likewise, the prevalence of tuberculosis, rickets and chronic infectious disease in nineteenth-century Britain can be presumed to have played a part in presentation. Evidence from Finnane (1981), reviewing pauper asylums in post-Famine Ireland, indicates that patients were 'chiefly affected with chronic disease', and even in 1914 'by far the largest number were found to be in a low state of bodily health' (p. 137). A comparison between the pauper clientele of the North Riding Asylum and the upper-middle class patients at The Retreat in York (Renvoize & Beveridge, 1989) showed an increased mortality rate in the former, due to physical ill-health.

Compared to a pauper population such ill-health would have been of lesser significance, particularly in relation to nutritional deficiency disorders, but the possibility of a number of cases being secondary to physical disease cannot be discounted. While wealth and plenty may have protected the average Ticehurst inmate from the worst ravages of poverty-related illness – thus supporting the view that a pauper asylum population may have been no less severely disturbed – it is still likely that chronic physical disorders were more prevalent than today. Such extreme states of mental illness as are described must also have affected attitudes as to the role of caring personnel. Not only did they have to attend to incoherent language and eccentric behaviour, but this was often associated with disordered bowel movements, various skin conditions, physical infirmity and other nursing needs. Washing, feeding, dressing and administering medicines accompanied 'moral' treatments and appropriate behavioural examples. Physical methods such as stomach pumps, mustard baths and electrical treatment would have made sense in such conditions.

Given such severity, physicality and recognizability, is it then surprising that the medical profession should have taken over the management of madness? Descriptions of delirium tremens, by Sutton in 1813, and the cerebral pathology of GPI, by Bayle in 1826, had reinforced the somaticist view earlier in the century. While the importance of 'moral treatment', as advocated by Tuke (1813) in his description of the Retreat at York, and the need for non-restraint, as stressed by Gardiner Hill (1838) and Conolly (1856), were dominant management methods, physical treatments continued to be used. The details of their range and effectiveness have yet to be adequately researched, and the apparently punitive role of shower baths, cathartics and blisterings has led to a considerable denunciation of mad-doctors by contemporary and modern authors. Alongside such criticism has grown the notion that a driving motive behind the rise of the asylums was the search for power and status by the newly emerging psychiatric profession (e.g. Scull, 1979; Busfield, 1986; Porter, 1987). By stressing the need for early asylum care and active physical treatment medical men have been seen as imposing a medical model on individuals who may merely have been socially deviant or harmlessly eccentric.

Yet the picture seen at grass-roots level in the Ticehurst Casebooks is much more one of powerlessness. Patients came and went, often at the whim of families, who would decide after a 'family meeting' not to pursue admission or would precipitately have their relative 'removed', possibly for economic reasons. Outcomes that were 'relieved' or 'improved' were much more typical than 'cured'. Despite all their accoutrements of measured walks, generous diets, numerous attendants and physical therapies, the Newingtons had to deal with constant disappointments. They and their attendants were assaulted and abused. They had to cope with the sordid business of nursing demented paralytics through months of increasing inanition and incontinence. A residuum of chronic incurables lived on in the asylum, playing cricket, attending concerts, going to the seaside, but not getting better. The public views of asylums, and asylum doctors were not much more than grudging, and the need for sheer practical energy, as evinced in the lifestyle of H. H. Newington (Obituary, 1917), must have been paramount.

A final, general, point also pertains to the medical role in asylums. For the symptoms and behaviour noted in the Casebooks, while sometimes given a descriptive diagnosis, such as 'acute mania', were often left to speak for themselves without any attempt at nosological clarification. This has a close parallel in the practices described at the York Retreat (Digby, 1985, p. 137), where 'during much of the second half of the nineteenth century, medical labelling of patients seems to have been honoured more in the breach than in the observance'. Apart from broad general terms like 'mania', 'melancholia' and 'dementia', and symptomatic phrases or words, e.g. 'delusions' or 'aural hallucinations', there was only a very limited attempt at diagnosis. For example, the contentious label 'moral insanity' was used for only three admissions in the 1845–90 period, and between 1890 and 1906 again only three times. In one case it was the basis for removal from the asylum. Likewise in the Casebook notes it is surprising when a diagnostic comment is actually made. For example, Mr R.S. was described as an example of 'insanity of adolescence', while Mr H.G. was deemed typical of 'chronic dementia'. But more often broad general terms were employed both in initial assessments of the mental state (e.g. 'depression with excitement') and in follow-up notes.

Those noted comments were often limited and practical, with few attempts at psychological speculation or aetiological concern. Such linguistic barrenness is a considerable contrast to the rich details of management and organization that made the asylum work. Yet this same emphasis on practical matters seems to have been a significant aspect of the views of contemporary alienists, critics of whom may have been puzzled by the discrepancy between theory and practice. Expecting asylum doctors and mental specialists to be learned philosophers of the mind, able to discuss mind–brain physiology and sophisticated diagnostic classifications, highbrow intellectuals would have been disappointed at the concentration on administration and physical approaches. The volumes of the *Journal of Mental Science* (*JMS*) were full of papers and discussions on ventilation, asylum design, and neuropathology, only sometimes leavened by Henry Maudsley's darker philosophizing. But the importance of the physician's personality, of the personnel attending the patients, and of the social networks thus provided – two out of three individuals encountered at Ticehurst during the day would have been non-lunatic – shines through every page of these Casebooks. Coping with the demands of the insane required skills more associated with army logistics than a university common-room.

RELIABILITY AND VALIDITY OF THE DATA

A key question in the examination of the Ticehurst Casebooks was the possibility of applying modern diagnoses to the available material. Since the essence of clinical psychiatry is the personal interview with a patient, some critics would at once denounce an approach made on the basis of notes alone. Yet there are clear and useful precedents for such retrospective analysis (e.g. Shepherd, 1957; Tsuang & Winokur, 1975) in modern research aimed at studying the course, genetics and outcome of schizophrenic and manic-depressive illnesses. Criteria have been developed, such as the Research Diagnostic Criteria (Spitzer *et al.* 1975) (RDC), used here alongside ICD-9 (Spitzer *et al.* 1978) that are specifically capable of giving a diagnosis within broad limits, based on either an interview or assessment of clinical notes. Provided sufficient details of mental and physical states are available, the process of reaching a clear diagnosis is straightforward. Interpreting terms such as 'ambivalence' or 'depression' is not required, since behaviours and time-courses are clearly delineated, and specific psychopathology, such as delusions, hallucinations or formal thought-disorder, is formally defined. Unlike the Present State Examination (PSE, Wing *et al.* 1974), no formal training is required, although checking reliability with other practitioners, as was done in this case, is regarded as a useful routine. In the final analysis the only absolute check on reliability would be another complete review of the Casebooks by experienced clinical and research psychiatrists. One of the strengths of the present investigation is that it can be repeated, *ad infinitum*, by psychiatrists of successive generations as well as by contemporaries. The material may well serve as a template for comparative diagnoses across many years.

As to the validity of the diagnoses *per se*, this investigation is not aimed at refining nosological boundaries. 'Few psychiatric disorders have yet been adequately validated' (Kendell, 1989) and broad acceptance of the clinical categories used in the RDC (and in ICD-9) is based on a realistic understanding of the present limits of psychiatric diagnoses. Compared to the sophisticated neuro-chemical understanding of many physical illnesses, mental diseases are much more poorly defined, often being symptom clusters as much as coherent entities. Nevertheless 'the development of disease constructs for certain mental disorders is meaningful if they provide at least an adequate explanation of the symptom clusters, the underlying pathological mechanisms and the course of the disorder' (Häfner, 1987). Such definitions also provide researchers with cohorts of significantly similar patients whose characteristics can be examined and compared with other groups in the search for causative factors and appropriate treatments. The diagnostic categories used in this study have been deliberately broadened out to the five groupings described in the Introduction and Results. Comprising 'schizophrenia', 'manic-depressive illness', 'neurotic disorders', 'organic disorders' and 'uncertain', they fulfil the bulk of a present-day hospital psychiatric caseload. Terms such as 'schizo-affective disorder' have also been used, and such a term certainly seemed the best description of several cases, but such subcategories were not really relevant to the purposes of this study, although interesting in themselves.

Specific examples of diagnoses are given in the Appendix. The details provided are a précis of the original notes; comments as to the factors contributing to the diagnosis are given as a brief summary of each case. In conditions defined by clear, positive symptoms it is not difficult to reach diagnostic decisions. Thus, in example No. 1 there are descriptions of her delusions, of her passivity experience of thought withdrawal (a combination of two first-rank symptoms), and of her persistent and increasing incoherence associated with 'grossly disorganized behaviour'. There is no evidence of manic-depressive symptoms and the time-course is prolonged. Such a cluster comprises a satisfactory diagnosis of schizophrenia as understood in research terms. More problematical are those cases lacking clear descriptions of symptoms, or lacking sufficient symptoms to clinch a psychotic

diagnosis. Thus, a Mrs J. S. has a number of unusual symptoms, such as suicidal ideas or possibly even true delusions, but the evidence is never quite hard enough for a diagnosis of major depressive disorder. Some analysts might contend that she was sufficiently 'agitated', 'suicidal', 'insomniac' and socially changed to fulfil the criteria, but the needs of this study dictated a bias towards scepticism and uncertainty rather than searching desperately for a clear diagnosis. A review of those cases deemed 'uncertain' (e.g. Appendix, example No. 3) might well increase the number of positive diagnoses, and certain characteristics of this group (e.g. length of stay, prevalence of movement disorder) link it to schizophrenia. Thus, Miss Mary Harvey (example No. 3) 'remains in one attitude for hours', uses 'bad language' and avoids 'all treatment and interference'. This might be seen as reflecting thought disorder and grossly disorganized behaviour, fulfilling criteria A-8 for schizophrenia (probable) in the RDC. However, in this case and many others the behavioural descriptions were regarded as lacking sufficient detail to allow extrapolation to an accepted diagnosis.

With regard to 'Organic' diagnoses, these could be guaranteed only by post-mortem findings. But evidence of overt physical symptoms or cognitive impairment was often convincing enough to accept cases into a broad category such as this. Cases include Mr E. S. (Casebook 6) and example No. 3 (Rev. A. B. – see Appendix). The former was admitted 'in a state of tremor', with 'skin damp', 'pulse 80', 'function of the liver greatly damaged' and 'memory clouded'. The latter evinced 'great loss of memory' – with an excellent example of short-term memory loss – had 'defective articulation', again with an example given, and a 'gait weak and unsteady'. He progressed to involuntary salivation, partial paralysis and difficulty in swallowing, all signs of neurological impairment. Both cases were described in terms used today, namely delirium tremens and general paralysis (of the insane), and the signs and symptoms accord with such diagnoses.

Post-mortems were intermittently performed and described in some detail; clear records exist for at least nine cases. Five of these had definite organic illnesses; curiously enough all were male, and the latter six had relatively brief periods of admission before death. In a minor way, therefore, the search for an underlying physico-pathological cause of disturbed behaviour was pursued, and a close watch for the development of physical signs was maintained. The reliability and validity of the diagnoses included in the organic category seem satisfactory and, as stated above, if anything this group was under-represented in the final figures.

It should be stressed that the process of reaching a diagnosis was reviewed twice. The initial reading of the Casebooks involved extracting phrases and terms from the notes such as were in any way relevant, whether positive or negative, to the final diagnosis. From this an initial diagnosis was reached. All diagnoses made during one session were subsequently reviewed at the next session, and again reviewed when all the summaries were analysed for aspects of other data concerning masturbation, symptoms, treatments, etc. In general, few changes emerged during this process. The second review was specifically aimed at rejecting diagnoses based on unclear or limited data and at increasing the proportion of 'uncertain' cases. In fact the occasional changes noted were in the opposite direction, because of previous failures to include significant symptoms.

STRENGTHS AND WEAKNESSES OF THE SOURCE MATERIAL

The use of contemporary Casebook notes, as opposed to published cases, in the historical analysis of mental illness is a relatively new departure. Outstanding examples include the work of Tomes on Thomas Kirkbride and the Pennsylvania Hospital for the Insane (Tomes, 1984), and Digby's study of the York Retreat 1796–1914 (Digby, 1985). This study has been more limited in that it has almost entirely confined itself to casebook material, attempting to focus on diagnostic issues rather than the broad social role of asylums. A key question must be the reliability of the medical notes as a true record of psychological and behavioural phenomena.

The format of the records may in itself bias the data, for an 'Order as to the Case Book' was laid down by the Commissioners in Lunacy. This required basic details of name, age, sex and mental status, descriptions of the physical state

and 'phenomena of mental disorder', particulars of the previous history, and a statement of changes in the patient's health and the remedies employed in treatment. Such demands were time-consuming and the need to provide suitable material may have led to an over-enthusiastic use of professional terms such as 'delusions'. This word is very common, and as often refers to unusual ideas that may have been true (e.g. about the possession of large sums of money) as to phenomena regarded as formally 'delusional' by modern standards. According to Fish (1974), 'the essence of the primary delusional experience is that a new meaning arises in connection with some other psychological event'. Mullen (1986) suggested that delusion 'involves abnormal beliefs that arise in the context of disturbed judgements and on occasion an altered experience of reality, such that it becomes a source of new and false meanings'. Nowhere in the casenotes are such definitions attempted, but often examples of delusional ideas are given, persistently, with details as to how they affected behaviour. Patients' own words are also used to describe such experiences, although it is uncertain to what extent these have been copied directly or quoted from memory. Numerous letters and drawings fill out such material.

The details of particular patients also vary. The earliest notes (in Casebook 1) are rudimentary and often brief, covering less than half a page, although there is considerable variation. Until the notes of Mrs E. (Casebook 2, admitted February 1851) are reached, insufficient detail is available for analysis in most cases. Thereafter a different order of description ensues, possibly due to the insistence of the Lunacy Commissioners (Mackenzie, 1986). Even so, there is much variation, which may arise from aspects of the patients themselves. Previous family and personal history would largely rely on having friends or family members available and willing to divulge such secrets. A disturbed individual might not be examined physically or questioned closely about his mental state. The more interesting phenomena may be written up in detail, selectively biasing diagnoses towards particular syndromes. Different resident medical officers might alter the details and language of description, producing case material representative of their nosological interest or previous experience rather than an objective account of phenomena. Training in psychological medicine was limited and variable during this period, and errors in assessment and diagnosis, as well as a mistaken use of technical terms, may have occurred.

It must also be remembered that these notes were written up for perusal by the Lunacy Commissioners. That was their initial purpose, although once a routine was established, once annotation became part and parcel of clinical practice, a less self-conscious tone may have emerged. The expectation of inspection may have altered, nevertheless, their content and detail. Statements and behaviour indicating insanity may have been embellished so as to conform with official notions of true mental illness. The beneficial effects of asylum care and treatment may have been over-stressed, and the use of the terms 'recovered' and 'relieved', for cases in which little objective change had been recorded, could reflect this need for justification. These two terms, and 'cured', accounted for 69% of those in Ticehurst for less than one year, 42·2% of those in for one to five years, and 6·7% of those in for more than five years. They may therefore merely be related to length of stay rather than any objective improvement. Certainly it behoves the modern assessor to be extremely sceptical as to the reality of such outcome terms.

However, such inherent tendencies for notes to conform to a stereotype, as required by the writer or those he was writing for, would have been counteracted by other forces. The Newingtons themselves stated that 'Hereditary predisposition is a hopelessly unknown quantity. We get in time to hear of a history in many cases which has been denied unblushingly on admission. With us mendacity is added in probably a greater degree to ignorance of family history than is usual in most institutions' (Medical Superintendents, 1901). Lacunae in the history of events leading up to admission would severely damage any aetiological thesis, as well as the validity of the contemporary, initial, diagnosis. To what extent such gaps were allowed to extend into the routine Ticehurst notes is uncertain. A number of applicant relatives remain anonymous. Families may have requested – but this is only speculative – that as limited a record as possible be kept of their relative's odd, or disgusting, or dangerous behaviour. The variable details of the notes certainly conforms to no set pattern, sparseness generally coinciding with length of stay and chronicity of illness. Some cases seem poorly described, others illustrated at exhaustive length. A number of routine phrases are employed, and there is a general tendency for increasing conformity during the 1870s and 1880s. The language thus remains unimaginative and descriptive, with limited use of technical jargon or theorizing.

A particular strength of the notes is the regular concern with basic biological functions. Appetite and weight, sleep, daytime activity, forms of speech, social interaction and modes of dress are constantly recorded in almost obsessive detail. Such factors are especially important in assessing manic-depressive disorders, where disturbances of sleep, eating, activity and social behaviour form part of the key criteria for reaching a diagnosis. As the century proceeded there was also increasing resort to numerical data. Instead of describing sleep or appetite as poor, definite numbers are given, of hours slept or of weight lost or gained. At least twenty outstanding instances of this form of measurement provided three examples in the 1860s, five in the 1870s and eleven in the 1880s. Formal pulse rates, temperature charts and nursing observations (as used today) did not come in until the early 1900s. While such data certainly enhanced a formal view of changing behaviour and physical state, again it may be selective in highlighting certain types of case, not least because it remained the exception.

Overall, though, it is probably reasonable to view the notes as defining some form of reality. There was an intrinsic need to create a true picture of a patient's state as a background for therapeutic achievement, legal information and clinical understanding. Many individual sets of handwriting are found, reflecting different viewpoints and levels of experience. Legibility, lack of erasures, and the completeness of the Casebooks as a body of information give no grounds for assuming any regular attempts at censorship or rearrangement of the material.

IMPLICATIONS OF DIAGNOSES

Bearing in mind these reservations as to the completeness and objectivity of the Ticehurst notes, on the whole it seems reasonable to accept their account of events in the absence, as yet, of any countervailing information. The process of retrospective diagnosis may be more contentious, but there seem sufficient precedents in modern and historical research to give it some validity. At the practical level it seems reasonable to assume that most psychiatrists would accept most of the diagnoses and most of the uncertainties. How then can this perspective usefully examine practices and patients in Victorian Sussex?

(A) 'Manic-depressive' and 'schizophrenic' groups

The most striking fact is the percentage of positive diagnoses for the cohort as a whole, as recorded in Table 1. Eliminating the 80 patients admitted before the fuller documentation of the 1850s, nearly 80% can be given a positive diagnosis: 41·7% seem to have manic-depressive illnesses, 26% schizophrenic and 15% organic. There is also considerable uniformity of diagnosis over time, particularly from 1860 onwards. The earlier, pre-1849, period is striking for the prevalence of uncertain diagnoses, largely due to lack of information, and the absolute lack of any clear-cut manic-depressive states. The unusually high proportion of neurotics (18%) in 1845–9 may contain some of these, limited data making a bias towards minor, as opposed to major, depressive disorder in the RDC. The lack of routine biological information (on appetite, sleep, etc.) was also certainly operative. By contrast, schizophrenic illnesses were only slightly reduced, since diagnosis rested upon detecting one or two positive symptoms rather than accumulating reliable behavioural information. It must also be remembered that 'in 1840 things with us appear to have become very dull, the place being filled up with hardy perennials', (Medical Superintendents, 1901) and that in 1852 Charles Newington died. It seems likely, therefore, that a distinct change in admission policy occurred after this period, particularly once the asylum had expanded to the 80 or so inmates described in 1901. From an average admission rate of about five per year until 1859, Ticehurst increases its turnover to over 11 per year in the early 1860s, and over 16 per year subsequently.

The diagnostic data give some insight into how this was achieved, namely an appropriate balance between the more chronic illnesses of the schizophrenic spectrum and the self-limiting ones associated with mania (modern) and depression. Once the 1855–9 quinquennium is reached, the diagnostic balance remains remarkably stable. Between a quarter and one-third of admissions were schizophrenic, between a third and a half were manic-depressive and about 5% seem to have had neurotic illnesses. The only major aberration is the 25% organic cases for 1865–9, largely composed of patients with GPI. The simultaneous introduction in Ticehurst of mustard treatment at this time may be related to a specific therapeutic strategy for the mania preceding paralysis. Such figures may even reflect a general upsurge in those seeking treatment for the disease itself, as part of the economic prosperity of the times. Given the differential diagnosis between mania secondary to GPI and 'manic-depressive' mania, it may merely have been due to clinical factors. In attempting to balance out the poor prognosis cases with a suitable leavening of apparently treatable affective disorders, the proprietors had to accept a degree of paralytic fall-out.

Of course, the process of admission itself may have had little to do with diagnostic factors. Among the Ticehurst material there is an unnumbered 'Casebook 1857–1873' which contains some details of those applying for places in the asylum. The information is limited and sketchy, but of 480 'Applications' recorded, 181 patients were admitted. Of another 189, no further comment was made, while 34 had some form of alternative care provided because of 'urgency' or the need for a more local resource. The remainder were either 'declined' by 'Dr. N' (25) or offered terms that were deemed 'too low' or 'unsuitable' (51). There was rarely any explanation for this. One potential patient was considered 'objectionable' because a relation was already 'in the Establishment', another sent elsewhere 'being a decided suicide', another refused 'under peculiar circumstances'. When admission was accepted, it usually happened without delay. For those clearly dated, 56% came in within a week, another 25% within a month and most of the rest within three months. In other words, there was a plentiful supply of customers who could be admitted quickly if accepted or rejected if deemed unsuitable. The proprietors – that is, the Drs Newington – had some choice in the matter.

Such inferences are supported by the data on length of stay and outcome in Tables 5 and 6. Those admitted for less than one year are predominantly manic-depressive (52·9 %), while the schizophrenic proportion is reduced to 17·5 %. Though nearly 10 years older on average, and more likely female, over half of the manic-depressives are deemed 'cured' or 'recovered'. The picture among the long-stay patients is reversed. Only 16·2 % are manic-depressive while 60 % are schizophrenic, and none are 'neurotic'. Even allowing for the fact that many discharges may have been due to economic, family or behavioural factors (e.g. persistent violence), there is a distinct trend in the relationship between diagnosis and length of stay.

To what extent, though, would a reasonable balance of patients have been important in running a private asylum such as Ticehurst? While a regular core of chronic inmates supplied a reliable income, it may have been important to the establishment's reputation and morale to have a number of cases leaving 'cured' and/or 'recovered'. The skill of the Newingtons may thus have been broadly prognostic, in that they were able to differentiate between those liable to recover and those liable to linger. Detailed classifications, using numerous subcategories, would not have been useful to them in this regard. They also seem to have accepted primarily psychotic pathology, thus the very small number of neurotics. This group seems also to have been unattractive in having an average-to-poor recovery rate – perhaps related to personality problems? – particularly if they stayed for more than a year, and in providing a number of irksome management problems.

(B) 'Organic' group

As stated above, this cohort, particularly those with GPI, may well have caused difficulties in the business of selecting a good prognosis clientele. Largely male, they had an appalling death rate, over 40 % dying within a year, and 74·2 % dying within 1–5 years. Recovery was almost entirely due to the alcohol-related conditions, such as delirium tremens, and the details of the slow, sordid decline into dementia of middle-aged men do not make for pleasant reading. As a group they are quite distinct in

terms of outcome and sex, reinforcing the view that hidden organic conditions were not a significant part of other cohorts.

(C) 'Indefinite' group

This group is small but tends to increase with increasing length of stay, comprising 7·5 % of the ' < 1 year' cohort, 10·3 % of the '1–5 years' cohort and 15·2 % of the 'five years and more' cohort. Such an increase is only matched by the schizophrenic group. It also shares with the schizophrenics a younger-than-average age (34·95 years) and a significant tendency to be single. In fact, it is the least married of all the groups, only 20 % overall being married compared to 28 % of the schizophrenics and 57 % of the manic-depressives. Its outcome profile is also relatively poor, approximating most nearly to the schizophrenics. If one also considers the data from Table 6, this group is very like the schizophrenics in terms of the percentages described as violent, having a movement disorder, and as masturbating. All of which points to the likelihood that most of the uncertain cases had schizophreniform illnesses, probably characterized by chronic behavioural and negative symptoms, and a more obvious defect state. Such an inference receives support from analysing the contemporary diagnostic terms used across the modern diagnostic groupings.

CONTEMPORARY DIAGNOSTIC TERMS USED AT TICEHURST

The business of diagnostic classification of mental disease flourished in the nineteenth century, as acknowledged with some scepticism by Bucknill & Tuke in their *Manual of Psychological Medicine* (Bucknill & Tuke, 1858). Chapter V, 'On The Definition of Insanity, and of Classification', opens with a quote from Dr Johnson concerning attempts to define poetry, 'namely, that such attempts at definition will only show the narrowness of the definer'. It was also admitted that 'very different arrangements have been made by different writers of the symptoms manifested of the insane' (p. 89); thus the conclusion as to 'placing before him [the student] little more than the typical forms of mental disease'. These are idiocy, dementia, delusional insanity, emotional insanity and mania, with the rider that 'all the above forms of

Mental Disorder may be complicated with General Paralysis, or with Epilepsy'.

Such groupings were significantly different from the principal forms of insanity according to the 1844 report of the Metropolitan Commissioners in Lunacy. Their headings were mania, dementia, melancholia, monomania, moral insanity, congenital idiocy, congenital imbecility, general paralysis of the insane and epilepsy. Of course, by the end of the century significant changes had occurred such that Clouston in his *Clinical Lectures on Mental Diseases* (Clouston, 1904, 6th edn) could give nineteen 'chief varieties' of insanity based on physiological causes (e.g. lactational insanity, alcoholic (and toxic) insanity), although his symptomatological classification had only eight major groups partly related to the earlier categories. There were many more subgroups, however, so that 'States of Mental Exaltation (Mania, Psychlampsia)' included simple, acute, delusional, chronic, ephemeral (mania transitoria) and homicidal mania (p. 10). Given that Hayes Newington trained at Edinburgh under Clouston, and was his first Senior Assistant Physician at Morningside (Obituary, 1917), it is reasonable to expect that diagnoses at Ticehurst in the 1870s and 1880s might reflect some of Clouston's terminology.

What influences, if any, affected the earlier period are more obscure. The language of Bucknill and Tuke, and the Lunacy Commission, cannot have gone unnoticed, especially since the latter 'commented regularly on defective medical casebooks in licensed houses, and on the inadequacy of certificates' (Hervey, 1987, p. 220).

Some details of the relationship between contemporary and modern diagnoses, over the four decennia between 1850 and 1889 are enumerated in Tables 2–4, and several general themes are apparent. Most striking is the variety and looseness of the terms, particularly with regard to the 'schizophrenia' group. There is also a progressive development towards a wider variety of categories and an interesting phase during the 1860s when about 20% of the patients simply were not given any admission diagnosis at all.

The least-coherent group is that fulfilling modern criteria for schizophrenia (Table 2). Acknowledged by Bleuler, in his seminal work,

as *The Group of Schizophrenias* (1950) (the emphasis is on the plurality of the term), schizophrenia 'is best considered as a syndrome that may cover several conditions' (Murray, 1986). At Ticehurst the term 'delusions' predominates overall, being used in nearly half of all the cases, but declines over time from 83·5% to 26·2% by the 1880s. 'Dementia' is little used – by contrast with the 'indefinite' group where it constitutes 12·9% of all diagnostic terms – and 'melancholia' and 'monomania' are similarly rare. The word 'hallucinations' comes to some significance by the 1880s, but the only other formal category that has any importance is mania, especially chronic mania in the 1870s and 1880s. Here the Cloustonian influence may be apparent, but overall only just over a third of all the cases (34·5%) have been allocated to an accepted diagnosis rather than a symptomatic term (e.g. 'aural hallucinations'). This is in clear contrast to the diagnoses made for both 'indefinite' and 'manic-depressive' categories, where 62·9% and 61·8% of the patients respectively have received a formal diagnosis. Such an inability to allocate cases now deemed broadly schizophrenic may reflect the variable symptoms of the syndrome and the resultant difficulties faced by Victorian private asylum keepers in agreeing on a diagnostic term. Able enough in assessing individual symptoms such as delusions or hallucinations, they may have lacked sufficiently large case-material (possibly via selective process – see below) to discern a syndromal pattern in the somewhat inchoate mass of presentations with which they had to deal.

However, when one is confronted with the more coherent manic-depressive disorders, a different picture emerges. While the term, 'delusions' still dominates the 1850s (see Table 4), it becomes less and less prominent and increasingly part of a descriptive phrase such as 'melancholia and delusions' or 'mania with delusions'. Melancholia and mania, especially 'acute' and 'subacute' mania, advance inexorably to over 80% of the diagnoses by the 1880s. Not only is there good agreement between nineteenth-century and modern usage of the terms, but coherence of diagnosis at Ticehurst is obvious. In a small way it is thus possible to watch the development of a clear diagnostic category that has survived largely unchanged to the present day. From being general terms defining over-activity and underactivity within the broad compass of insanity, melancholia and mania become increasingly mood-specific disorders distinct from other functional psychoses. The separation emerges perhaps via the prefixes 'acute' and 'chronic', the latter used only twice in the 'manic-depressive' group but fourteen times in that of 'schizophrenia'. Furthermore, alternative diagnostic language is rarely required, although a subclassification using prefixes such as 'puerperal', 'paroxysmal' and 'senile' is attempted.

Such an overall trend towards agreement and clarity, in contrast to the uncertainties within the 'schizophrenia' group, may well be a reflection of a selective admission policy as suggested earlier. The relationship between diagnosis and asylum management can therefore be seen as dynamic and coherent rather than casual. It might also suggest that the process of honing diagnostic clarity had a strong social pressure behind it. To project an asylum with a good record of 'cured' or 'recovered' patients it was important to know your clientele and the prognosis of the conditions you accepted. Commenting on private asylum care in 1862, Wraxall wrote, 'for as the demands for admission are generally in excess of the accommodation, it is naturally to the interest of the proprietors to discharge a large annual number, and thus maintain the good character of their houses'. Unlike a large public asylum in which admission was not under control of the doctors (e.g. Hunter & MacAlpine, 1974, p. 17; Cochrane, 1988), or in which they acquiesced in a diagnosis made outside the institution (Dwyer, 1987, p. 117), private establishments were able to use medical criteria more purposefully in the selection and management of patients. Of course, it may be that the proportion of diagnoses seen in Ticehurst simply reflected admissions as a whole in Victorian England, but we lack the evidence at present to make such an assumption.

Comments need also to be made concerning the lesser categories, although the numbers involved are few. Those with an 'indefinite' diagnosis today show no particular consistency of contemporary diagnosis, although there is a trend towards the use of the term 'mania'. This conforms to the pattern of the 'schizophrenia' and 'manic-depressive' groups, with a total

usage (29·6%) that falls between the 21·8% of the former and the 33% of the latter. The 'indefinites' do differ significantly in having a higher rate of 'dementia' (12·9%) and in being more often given no diagnosis at all (11·1%). They also tend to be less often described with the term 'delusions', in contrast to all other categories. Thus 48·6% of 'schizophrenics', 46·2% of 'neurotics', 27·8% of 'manic-depressives' and 26·9% of 'organics' are given this label, but only 18·5% (10 out of the 54) of 'indefinites'. Two of the moral insanity cases come into this modern category and even melancholia is poorly represented, comprising just 7·4% of the total. The picture is one lacking in positive symptoms and lacking in any sense of contemporary diagnostic coherence. Linked with other factors associated with this group, such as movement disorder and violence, a significant proportion would most likely have a defect-state characteristic of chronic schizophrenia (Wing, 1961). Reinforcing this inference is the prevalence of characteristic negative symptoms (poverty of speech, social withdrawal, flattening of affect) among this cohort. The descriptive results include a number of typical cases wherein terms such as 'incoherence', 'vegetative', 'solitary' and 'torpid' abound.

The process of diagnosis, as a whole, and as seen in the light of modern categories, does not seem to have been very precise or discussed in much detail. The major concern (from the 1860s onwards) elicited from the notes was whether or not an individual with obvious manic symptoms had significant neurological signs. Inequality of pupils, tremulousness of the tongue, a tottering gait, were carefully looked for and described with varying degrees of certainty. The phrase 'No symptoms of epilepsy or paralysis', or variants thereof, came into routine use. But this attention to physical signs seems to have been aimed primarily at assessing prognosis regardless of the specific diagnostic classification. And given that over 40% of the post-1850 cases were manic-depressives, the impact of GPI on the composition of private asylum inmates takes on a particular significance. The equivalence of Victorian and modern versions of mania is striking, contrasts with the ubiquity of terms for other conditions, and suggests that an expertise in such diagnosis had a major impact on the practices then prevalent. Here was a group that could recover fully or slide into dementia and death. From the treatment perspective, new drugs, mustard baths, electricity and hydro-therapy, vigorous physical exercise and dietary innovations could not be ignored once they had been associated with several recoveries.

Such recoverability not only led to the early establishment of a robust, empirically derived diagnostic category, but highlights the relative lack of interest in other forms of psychiatric illness. Whether these were called 'dementia', 'chronic mania', 'delusions with hallucinations' or 'monomania' made no difference whatsoever. Whether dying or recovering, there was no obvious commercial or professional impetus towards improving diagnosis or innovating treatments. Such illnesses, described by Clouston (1888) as 'the great lowering agency in our asylums', provided a regular clientele for both public and private establishments. Their gath-ering in the large public asylums is prefigured in the outcomes recorded for those with 'schizo-phrenia' in Ticehurst, many of whom are transferred down the social ladder to less lavish places. Unlike the public asylums, however, 'the private mad-house keeper as speculative trades-man' (Parry-Jones, 1972) could not afford to let his establishment silt up with chronic incurables. To quote Parry-Jones (1972, pp. 84–90) again, 'continued success...depended to a large extent on the personal reputation of the proprietor and the public confidence he held'. Such reputations required close control of the selection and management of clientele, and a strongly practical streak. The methods by which the Newingtons organized their establishment, selecting and training their own attendants, inventing a machine for clocking in and out of work, designing measured walks in the grounds, using their own version of the stomach-pump, all reflect such a pragmatic approach (MacKenzie, 1986). The relationship between diagnostic terms, behaviour, and management can be further illustrated by looking at a small group of patients to which the term 'hysteria' (or 'hysteri-cal') was applied. Not only has this label been viewed with considerable scepticism by modern commentators (e.g. Showalter, 1985), but it also seems to have had little predictive power in Ticehurst. It reinforces the view that diagnosis *per se* was unimportant in running the asylum.

USE OF 'HYSTERIA', 'HYSTERICAL MANIA' AND RELATED TERMS

At least 16 cases were formally labelled as hysterical, although Table 9 also contains details of Mrs H.U. (admitted February 1866, re-admitted April 1867), who was diagnosed as 'nymphomania' and subsequently as 'eroto-mania'. This was presumably because of her 'lascivious expression' and 'attitude to the opposite sex' as noted in her first admission, and 'the lecherous look and...much erotic impulse and tendency' of her readmission. The term 'hysterical' was also used for other cases in the notes when describing isolated facets of be-haviour, but its contemporary meaning can best be understood by reviewing these 18 labelled cases. Furthermore, in nearly all instances the phrase was 'hysterical *mania*', the straight-forward diagnosis 'hysteria' never being used in isolation. One case was described as 'mania with hysteria', and another was given no diagnosis, but the term 'hysteria', in brackets, was appended, possibly later. In all, just under 3 % of the admissions to Ticehurst (18/601) were formally given this category, so it does not comprise a very large part of the clientele.

The general features of this group are of interest. They are, of course, all women, with an average age of 34·25 years, which is considerably younger than the average (42·72 years) for Ticehurst. Only four stay for more than 16 months, and three of these have an 'indefinite' modern diagnosis. There is a considerable degree of violence recorded (in eight out of 16 patients – two patients had two admissions) and only five patients (seven admissions) were discharged as 'cured/recovered'. Although including all five of the modern diagnostic categories, there is a considerable increase, in percentage terms, of the 'neurotic' group, with compensatory de-creases in the 'organic' and 'schizophrenia' groups. The numbers are small and should not be analysed too far, but the picture is not especially coherent and the outcome was not very promising. Good recovery was largely confined to those with an RDC diagnosis of 'mania' (five out of seven cases); conversely, only one of the mania diagnoses did not achieve such an outcome, and she was only in the asylum for two months. This group therefore seems to be rather diverse in a number of ways,

Table 9. *Cases in Ticehurst diagnosed 'hysterical mania' (HM) or hysteria (H) and related terms*
1850–1890

Case no.	Date	Age*	Sex	Marital status†	Length of stay (months)‡	Violence or restraint	Outcome§	Masturbation	Contemporary diagnosis	Modern diagnosis‖
147	1862	47	F	S	9	V	Cured	−	HM	Mania
172	1864	48	F	S	1	·	Cured	−	HM	Mania
177	1864	24	F	S	48	V	Unimproved	+	HM	?
197	1865	27	F	S	120	V & R	Not improved	+	Mania + H	?
201	1866	54	F	W	2	·	(Relieved)	−	HM	Minor depression
202	1866	28	F	M	9	·	Recovered	−	Nymphomania	?
220	1867	29	F	M	7	R	Improved	−	Erotomania	Mania
229	1867	20	F	S	10	V	Relieved	+	HM + hallucinations	Schizophrenia
263	1869	22	F	S	216	·	Died	−	· (hysteria)	?
318	1873	28	F	S	1	·	Relieved	−	HM + religious delusions	Minor depression
409	1879	40	F	M	15	·	Relieved	−	HM + delusions	Minor depression
419	1880	43	F	S	3	·	Cured	−	HM	Organic
438	1880	42	F	M	3	·	Died	−	HM + delusions	Minor depression
462	1882	40	F	S	16	V	Recovered	−	HM	Mania
571	1888	36	F	M	1	·	Recovered	−	H insanity	Mania
577	1889	28	F	S	44	V	Relieved	+	HM	Schizophrenia
588	1889	37	F	S	5	V	Discharged	−	HM	Schizophrenia
590	1889	31	F	M	2	·	Discharged	−	HM	Mania

* Average age 34·25 years.   † Single 11, married 7.   ‡ Length of stay > 16 months = 4.   § Cured/recovered 7, died 2.   ‖ Mania 6 (33 %), neurotic 4 (22·2 %).

linked by a form of behaviour, deemed to be hysterical, rather than by a perception of nosological similarity.

The nature of this behaviour, as described in the notes, seems to be that it did not conform to the true severity or expected symptoms of the disease. Patient F.H. (Nos. 147 and 172) was described as 'wayward', 'capricious' and 'fanciful'; E.A. (No. 177) was 'wayward' and 'obstinate'; G.S. (No. 197) did 'the opposite of what she was required to do', 'endeavoured to make herself sick' and showed 'an intense desire to romp and turn head over heels'. Her case was 'clearly one of hysterical mania and probably associated with ovarian irritation'. Patient F.E. (No. 201) 'pretends to be unconscious', complained of 'imaginary ailments' and was apparently 'addicted to complaining and mischiefmaking'. Patient G.D. (No. 409) constantly begged for chloroform ('Chloroform me, why will you not give me chloroform – I am in burning pain all over') and complained of insomnia, yet had 'good nights with only coloured draughts' of placebo medication and was 'discontented with everyone'. (This case is strongly reminiscent of a patient who 'inhaled a great deal of chloroform' in Kraepelin's outline

(Defendorf, 1902) of hysterical insanity, p. 249). Patient R.G. (No. 462) had 'innumerable whims and fancies', was 'fond of holding the doctor's hand' and 'very amorous in her conduct', and A.H. (No. 590) was 'laughing and crying' and saw 'things which alter in form and colour'.

Not uncommonly, such behaviour was accompanied by impulsive acts or various forms of fit. Patient F.S. (No. 577) intermittently went 'rigid' or 'stiff'; R.G. (No. 462) complained of 'fainting' attacks; E.H. (No. 419) went into a 'semi-unconscious state' from which it was 'difficult to be roused', and the differential diagnosis, between hysteria or 'cerebral irritation', was discussed. Patient E.A. (No. 177) was reported as having had 'slight attacks of an epileptoid character (not observed in the Establishment)', while F.H. (No. 147) had '2 slight epileptic seizures' a week before a morning (9.30 to 12.30) of apparently full-blown epilepsy, during which her 'seizures were very violent'. 'I never saw worse in female…12 leeches were applied to the temple and below the ears', reported the MO, yet the treatment relieved her and no further epileptic episodes were reported, although 'paroxysms of violence coming on without warning' did occur. Patient J.T. (No.

229) also went into 'fits of hysterical transport and rapture', a 'state bordering on a trance' and even a 'transitory cataleptic condition'. Screaming – 'a severe attack of hysterics yesterday – the screams were awful', – masturbation, in at least four cases, and unusual forms of violence (e.g. trying to bite off an attendant's nose) were also characteristic behaviours.

Yet the overall picture does not contrast significantly with the general behaviours, symptoms and management practices described for the patients in general. No special treatments were employed. No particular moralizing phrase or tone of voice was apparent. Terms like 'delusions', 'melancholia' or 'dementia' were used to describe aspects of the cases in the follow-on notes. In general, these 'hysterical' patients were younger women, who stayed in for a relatively short admission period, whose behaviour was a little more extravagant than seems to have been expected from the underlying symptoms, and who did not seem to respond very well to the therapeutic regime of Ticehurst. Some were clearly psychotic, at least half were overtly violent. They seem to indicate, if anything, a considerable uncertainty as to the use of the hysterical diagnosis by the Ticehurst physicians. The term did not predict a particular outcome, did not initiate a particular treatment and did not conform to any broad, modern, diagnostic group. There was a close relationship with what we today might call 'neurological' disturbance, as witness the faints and seizures recorded in several cases, but hysteria in itself did not seem to be recognized as primarily a form of insanity. Certainly, there is no evidence in the Ticehurst Casebooks that rich young women, diagnosed as hysterical, formed a significant part of the workload or were considered to be such. Nor is this view contradicted by subsequent, post-1890 practice, since only three more cases of hysterical mania were admitted up to 1906.

Such an absence from a busy private asylum is not surprising given the physicality of the term as used by contemporary practitioners. Bucknill & Tuke (1858) state quite flatly, 'Hysteria is not insanity. But there is a form of mental disease in which aggravated hysteria constitutes a prominent symptom.' They went on to delineate hysteria as affecting 'the female sex almost exclusively'; as 'characterized by sudden

attacks', and as having 'the globus hystericus, a facial expression better known than described, and attacks of partial or complete unconsciousness, convulsions, spasms and even lock-jaw' (p. 168). By 1874 they were even expressing doubt as to whether 'Hysterical Insanity is a frequent type form'. In 1904 Clouston described 'insanity engrafted on Hysteria', and wrote that 'typical hysteria, pure and simple is now recognized ... to have a mental complication.' However, 'these mental symptoms, not forming the chief features of the disease ... were not till lately reckoned as being of the nature of technical insanity, at least among the rich.' He admitted that 'such patients are rare in asylums' and that the 'usual type of case classified as hysterical insanity consists of mania or melancholia in a young woman with one or more of the following characteristics well-marked ...'. Among these characteristic symptoms Clouston included 'feigned bodily illness ...', 'marked erotic symptoms ... hysterical convulsions, a morbid waywardness or ostentatious and real attempts at suicide'. He also wrote that 'hysterical symptoms are exceedingly apt to occur in the insanities of puberty and adolescence in women, and ... the habit of masturbation is common', stressing the difficulties of classifying such cases correctly. To the modern clinician such problems are exemplified by reading what he describes as a characteristic letter of a maniacal hysterical girl, a letter (p. 534) exhibiting grandiose delusions, flight of ideas and the typical symptom pattern of RDC mania!

Viewing his comments in the light of the Ticehurst material, there is a considerable diagnostic and descriptive consensus. Insanity is deemed mania or melancholia, and management is based upon this primary diagnosis, while hysterical behaviours merely colour in the presentation. Such usage may reflect views of womanhood and attitudes towards disturbed females, but this is a secondary phenomenon and does not seem to have been of significance in admission procedures. If anything, the brief length of stay, often poor outcome and distressing, disturbed behaviours made hysterical clients unwelcome guests at Ticehurst. It is unlikely that other private asylums would have had a significantly different approach, although specialism in managing such cases may have informed individual establishments or physicians. It should also be noted that these cases largely preceded the great age (the 1890s) of hysteria as more than an adjectival term. Nevertheless, the evidence points to such 'hysterics' as exceptional (thus celebrated) rather than typical, and further research is needed to clarify their numbers in asylum and medical practice.

SYMPTOMS – DELUSIONS AND HALLUCINATIONS

The prevalence of the terms 'delusions' and 'hallucinations' has been outlined in the Results. They are a hallmark of diagnosis and are constantly used in the routine Casebooks to describe day-to-day phenomena of patients' mental states. Broadly speaking, it seems that delusions were the key symptom of insanity, the *sine qua non* of many admissions, the marker of a sufficient severity of mental illness. Hallucinations on the other hand seem to have been more related to the course and outcome of the admission, their development seen as predictive of chronicity rather than indicating any particular level of severity. The relationship between these terms and the modern diagnosis of schizophrenia is apparent from Table 2. Not only were nearly 50% of these cases called 'delusions' (or delusional) but the increasing use of the term 'hallucinations', up to 16·7% by the 1880s, is in marked contrast to all the other modern categories where it was never used at all as a primary diagnosis. In a small way, then, the rudiments of the modern diagnosis seem to be emerging from the varied terminology of the mid-nineteenth century. Yet at least 21% of the whole cohort, from the 1840s to 1890, seem to have had hallucinatory experiences. Why, therefore, was the term used relatively scarcely in describing the diagnosis? It is as if the presence of hallucinations during an acute illness was a rather routine, and therefore not a distinctive, event.

Certainly the contemporary literature of psychopathology, from Esquirol (1845) to Clouston (1904), indicates a widespread acceptance of the importance of hallucinations, but equally a perception that they were not confined to insanity nor even to one particular form of mental disorder. Esquirol wrote of hallucinations as 'a cerebral or mental phenomenon',

'occurring independently of the senses, and consisting of external impressions which the patient believes he experiences, although there is no external agent acting on the senses'. He contrasted them with illusions, wherein 'the sensibility of the nervous extremities is altered; it is exalted, enfeebled or perverted; the senses are active, and actual impressions solicit the reaction of the brain'. The influential de Boismont (1859) quoted Esquirol and similarly defined an hallucination 'as the perception of the sensible signs of the idea; and an illusion as the false appreciation of real sensations' (p. 19). Yet Esquirol 'proposed the word hallucination as having no determinate signification, and as adapted, consequently, to all the varieties of delirium which suppose the presence of an object', while de Boismont carefully described 'Hallucinations co-existing with sanity' in his second chapter, and also associated them with a wide variety of diseases and causes. Bucknill & Tuke (1858) stressed this distinction (p. 142) between physiological and pathological hallucinations, quoting de Boismont that thereby one 'leaves on their pedestal the statues of illustrious men, whom some would wish to throw down into the abyss of insanity'. Encouraging the reader 'not to forget that hallucinations may exist without insanity', they quoted the experiences of Samuel Johnson and Napoleon Bonaparte and give a considerable list of conditions in which they may occur.

Later British writers, such as Maudsley (1895) and Clouston (1904), also discussed hallucinations, but their comments were limited. To Maudsley they were 'not uncommon features of melancholia, especially in its acute forms' (p. 224), while Clouston reckoned 'certain cases of mania are greatly characterised by the prevalence of hallucinations', and felt that they (along with other similar symptoms) were 'explained by the theory of the morbid excitation of Ferrier's and Hitzig's localised centres in the cortex of the brain' (p. 164). Both saw them as of 'bad prognostic import', reflecting comments made by the earlier writers quoted in Bucknill & Tuke (e.g. 'their presence was observed, by Esquirol, to be little favourable to the cure of insanity' (p. 152)).

Delusions were generally given much more prominence, whole sections being devoted to them by Bucknill & Tuke (1858 – Of Delusional

Insanity, p. 130), Forbes Winslow (1866 – Stage of Aberration, pp. 190–205) and Clouston (1904 – States of Fixed and Limited Delusion, pp. 249–277). Nor were these notions of delusion significantly different from modern definitions. Thus 'By delusion we do not mean an exaggerated self-depreciation, or an excessive sensibility to the supposed neglect of friends... but... an intellectual error, caused by the pathological condition of the mind, and displaying itself in false sensation, perception, or conception...' (Bucknill & Tuke, 1858). Clouston (1904) defined an 'insane delusion' as 'a belief in something that would be incredible to people of the same class, education, or race as the person who expresses it, the belief persisting in spite of proof to the contrary, this resulting from diseased working of the brain convolutions'. Modern definitions elaborate upon these but share a core of identity. Thus, Kräupl-Taylor (1979) summarizes psychotic delusion as 'an absolute conviction of the truth of a proposition which is idiosyncratic, ego-involved, incorrigible, and often preoccupying'. Mullen (1986) stresses five key characteristics, including: '(1) They are held with absolute conviction and are experienced as self-evident reality...; (2) They are not amenable to reason nor modifiable by experience; (3) They are experienced as of great personal significance; (4) Their content is often fantastic or at the very least inherently unlikely; (5) They consist of convictions which are highly personal and idiosyncratic which are not likely to be shared even by those of very similar social and cultural backgrounds' (p. 17). Such characteristics were not always fulfilled by the delusions described at Ticehurst, but the fuller examples seem quite satisfactory. An increasing elaboration of description also parallels a decline in the use of the term 'delusions' as a primary diagnosis, and a limited increase in the use of the phrase 'aural (or auditory) hallucinations'.

An overall view of these changes, as seen through the diagnostic divisions of modern criteria, hints at several clues concerning the development of the concept of schizophrenia. Because while it is clear that the condition embraced by RDC existed in a remarkably similar form in the second half of the nineteenth century, it is also likely that it was less distinctive amid other contemporary psychopathology.

Hallucinations were apparently commonplace across a gamut of physical and mental diseases, and amongst a host of individuals and conditions not seen as diseased. They begin to emerge in the Ticehurst notes as a phenomenon worth detailing and using for diagnosis, but until the tide of paralytic, febrile, nutritional and other causes had gone down they could not be regarded as a particularly distinctive marker. They also shared with delusions a much more prominent place among the symptoms of what is now termed manic-depressive illness, since such disorders in the nineteenth century were more severe, often psychotic, and again complicated by paralytic illness (GPI). It should not therefore be seen as puzzling that Victorian alienists in England did not seem to make many significant diagnostic advances. Beset by a wide range of conditions, with often indistinguishable symptoms, their attention to diet, physical care and protection from harm would have enhanced chronicity without clarifying nosological entities. On the other hand, this very process may have played a role in the Kraepelinian analysis that emerged towards the end of the century. Because this was based on a systematic examination of the course of mental illness as much as the symptoms, a task requiring the prolonged asylum care of numerous patients, dementia praecox or schizophrenia may be said to have been conceived by the asylum movement. There is no evidence from Ticehurst that schizophrenic patients became an increasing proportion of the clientele, but there is a growing recognition of a chronically deluded and/or hallucinated cohort that did not die and did not get better. The difference between the bald 1845 phrase 'labouring under delusions' and one of Hayes Newington's detailed mental state assessments of 1886 (see Appendix) exemplifies this process.

It is also noteworthy that specific forms of disorder, such as Capgras or Cotard's syndrome, the various types of thought disturbance and passivity experience outlined in the RDC, and aspects of behaviours such as negativism were described rather than classified. That they are present seems undeniable, but most seem to have been subsumed under the broader notions of 'delusions' and 'impulse'. As noted earlier, the sheer practical task of looking after such a disturbed group of patients may not have promoted inquisitive thinking into the understanding of psychopathology. Much more thought seems to have gone into the organized coping with violence, masturbation and negative behaviour.

MOVEMENT DISORDERS

Perhaps one of the most unexpected findings in this study was the high prevalence of various forms of disordered movement, unusual postures and typical 'catatonic' phenomena. As outlined in Table 6, patients showing these characteristics had a particular diagnostic profile. Furthermore, not only did they, in over half the cases, tend to stay for more than five years, but their prognosis was very poor. Less than one in five was described as 'relieved' or 'recovered', and most of those thus categorized (10 out of 14) left within a year of admission. Their tendency to violence, other psychopathology, single status and a schizophrenic or indefinite diagnosis also marks them out as being a core group of difficult-to-manage patients with severe illnesses. It is difficult, in fact, to avoid the conclusion that many of the 'indefinite' group had a similar condition to those given a schizophrenic diagnosis since the lack of movement disorder in other groups is so striking.

It is of note that the face and arms were predominantly affected and the terms 'grimace', 'fidget' and 'jerky' were the common descriptions. Given that over a quarter of the whole schizophrenic cohort was thus affected, it seems likely that the phenomena were very like those associated with tardive dyskinesia. Since terms such as 'restlessness' and 'agitation', both of which were commonplace in the Casebooks, were not deemed sufficiently specific to classify the relevant patient as having a movement/posture disorder, it is likely that the prevalence (of 28 % among the schizophrenics) is an underestimate. Whatever the exact figure, it very nicely matches the 20–40 % range of prevalence given in many studies of tardive dyskinesia (Kennedy *et al.* 1971). Since the Ticehurst cohort was largely a long-stay one, the relationship between length of illness and the development of movement disorder seems similar to that underlying the choice of the word 'tardive' (i.e. of delayed onset) in the modern condition. All of

which seems to indicate that dyskinesia, of some form, is an intrinsic sign of chronic schizophrenic illness. Alternative hypotheses would be that the medication at Ticehurst included agents having similar properties to modern neuroleptic drugs, or that this cohort has been falsely diagnosed and in fact consisted of patients suffering from neurological disorders. The former is unacceptable given the drugs prescribed; the latter is contradicted by the lack of such signs of dyskinesia among the known organic group (who often had GPI, a disorder causing widespread and various cerebral and neurological damage). The very persistence of the symptoms, and the routine nature of their description, makes it unlikely that acute or sub-acute chorea, due to infection or tumours for example, is the true basis for the disorders.

That grimacing, posturing and such a range of unusual movements was described should really come as no surprise, given the traditional description of dementia praecox, by Emil Kraepelin. He included 'making faces or grimacing and the fine muscular twitching in the face' as important symptoms, and also described a range of impulsive actions, postures and 'catalepsy' as typical of the illness (Kraepelin, 1913, p. 24). Likewise Clouston (1904), though rather dismissive of the Kraepelinian concept, did mention that 'in many forms of insanity there are choreiform and rhythmical movements that may be called ideomotor'. He cited a case of 'excited melancholia...who makes the most extraordinary choreiform faces and grimaces in a sort of automatic unthinking way', and went on to state that 'this sort of movement is common among the insane, and I look on it as being in many of them closely allied to chorea' (p. 505). Nor was this merely a turn-of-the-century phenomenon. Griesinger (1867) included a section on the 'Elementary Disorders of Movement' (p. 104) and distinguished 'partial or general convulsive states' from those due to paralysis. He wrote: 'the persistent automatic grimacing...painful convulsions of the muscles of the neck – those confused convulsive movements of the extremities which cause the patient often to walk irregularly...are all phenomena of serious signification, and their contrivance usually indicates a transition to the state of incurability'. Such textbook descriptions may have been forgotten or viewed as exceptional cases, but the prevalence figures available from Ticehurst confirm those authors' insistence that dyskinesia was commonplace in the pre-neuroleptic era.

Interestingly, the modern literature seems to be moving towards just such a view, despite the present-day teaching that insists tardive dyskinesia is a side-effect of anti-psychotic medication. Thus, Stahl (1986) insisted that 'the pre-eminent challenge in the field of tardive dyskinesia research is to discover an antipsychotic drug which does not cause tardive dyskinesia'. Yet Owens *et al.* (1982) studied 411 hospitalized patients with chronic schizophrenia, including 47 never exposed to neuroleptic medication, because of an unusual psycho-dynamic and family-orientated approach in one section of the hospital. Their conclusion was that spontaneous involuntary disorders of movement can be a feature of severe, chronic schizophrenia unmodified by neuroleptic drugs. Likewise Waddington (1987), in a detailed review, suggested it was 'extremely difficult to demonstrate any general relationship between increasing drug exposure and the emergence of the syndrome', yet pointed to a 'striking consistency in the association' with cognitive dysfunction and negative symptoms. Accepting that 'recourse to the historical literature, from the pre-neuroleptic era, offers little quantitative guidance in the absence of systematic studies', he supported the findings of Rogers (1985) 'that mental and motor disorder' might 'both be an expression of a unitary cerebral disorder', and concluded that neuroleptic treatment 'interacts, in some as yet unknown way...to hasten the appearance of dyskinetic movements in individuals with the greater likelihood of ultimately having such movements spontaneously as cerebral deterioration proceeds'. In a small, but important, way the Ticehurst findings provide unvarnished, quantitative evidence supporting the intrinsic nature of dyskinesia in schizophrenia, and the relationship with longevity of illness.

An interesting sideline to this discussion is the work of Hunter *et al.* (1964), who were among the earliest authors to comment on this 'new syndrome' apparently attributable to phenothiazines. Yet they admitted that 'the agitation and restlessness of these patients and their obvious distress may be mistaken for mani-festations of the illness' (for example, psychotic mannerisms and stereotypes) and described a cohort all of whom were definitely 'brain-damaged'. Given Hunter's outstanding contribution to psychiatric history and detailed acquaintance with primary sources, it seems strange that he should have so readily differentiated tardive dyskinesia as a drug-induced phenomenon, particularly when in *Psychiatry for the Poor* (Hunter & MacAlpine, 1974) there is detailed comment on movement and posture disorder. In fact, when discussing long-stay patients they wrote that 'the usual story is that they came in with an abnormal mental state and developed an abnormal motor state', which included 'abnormal movements from tremor to choreoathetosis or a mixture of both, from simple facial and respiratory tics including hemispasm and torticollis to complex grimaces and mannerisms' (p. 255). Unlike the present study, Hunter *et al.*'s work at Friern was based largely on Annual Reports, the casenotes being usually too sparse – one line written up annually in the examples given – to provide a pervasive picture of disorder. This may have obscured clinical details or it may be that they changed their position on tardive dyskinesia given that the historical study was written some years later. In fact, this rather puzzling discrepancy may be seen as an excellent illustration of the urgent need for modern psychiatrists to research their clinical history, in particular the manifestations of unmodified, chronic schizophrenic illness.

MASTURBATION

Masturbation, or self-abuse, became an act of increasing concern to the Ticehurst physicians as the century progressed. The associations with a 'schizophrenic' and 'indefinite' diagnosis (see Table 6) enhance the likely synonymity of these conditions – supporting the 'movement disorder' evidence – and give the modern diagnostician an insight into the concept of 'masturbational insanity'. Stressed by Skae (1863) and Maudsley (1868), especially, as a significant cause of mental disease, masturbation was also seen as a sign of illness and created a wide range of treatment approaches.

It is also worth considering the relationship with violent behaviour and movement disorder and the broadening range of behaviours and symptoms attributed to self-abuse/mastur-bation. These included dyspepsia, shrivelled testicles, facial appearances (especially of tired-ness), restlessness, irritability and depression. The reasons behind this increasing attribution of disorder have been ably analysed by Edward Hare (Hare, 1962), who suggested that the impact of conservatism, 'under the guises of authority and morality', the poverty of scep-ticism (i.e. 'in medicine any hypothesis is better than none') and certain fallacies of reasoning (e.g. 'the biased sample', 'the false analogy', 'the therapeutic fallacy') were the key factors behind the persistence of the masturbatory hypothesis. None of this is contradicted by the Ticehurst material, which portrays an increasing, and increasingly distinct, group of patients who are seen to masturbate, who indulge in odd and often unpleasant behaviours, who are chron-ically or severely deranged, and for whom certain physical treatments are justified therefore as appropriate. There is often a moral tone to the medical statements about them (e.g. 'bad habit', 'dirty', 'disgusting'), yet the severity and physi-cality of the conditions seem to provide a justification and a rationale for medical therapy. Even the most extreme treatments were regarded as relatively benign in their effects compared to the apparently dreadful consequences of un-checked masturbation.

On a broader perspective, this exercise of a masturbatory hypothesis, clinical experience and nosological organization is one mark of the end of 'moral therapy' as the dominant therapeutic approach of nineteenth-century psychiatry. 'Moral' treatment had provided some of the impetus for building asylums, but the increasing size of such establishments in the public sector, their silting up with incurable, chronic, cases and the thrusts of neuropathological research and clinical acumen, seem to have promoted alternative theories and treatments. Moral ther-apy was not apparently effective, in particular when used on the demented and disinhibited clientele that is seen in the Ticehurst cohort. Despite their gallimaufry of resources, such as attendants behaving like 'body servants or valets' and 'knowing how to speak to gentle-men', pleasant walks and gardens, 'theatrical and other entertainments' and a band playing 'twice a week all the year round', the Newingtons were 'ready to apply any remedies that suggest themselves as being likely to benefit the case' (Medical Superintendents, 1901). Their use of blistering agents, pessaries and forms of restraint seems to belie their 1901 insistence that they depended 'mostly upon the exercise of common sense and the moral atmosphere that has been formed around us in the course of the long existence of the Institution'.

Of course, it is difficult to be certain as to how closely they followed the dominant theories or changes in therapeutic fashion. H. H. Newington, as Treasurer of the MPA from 1894 to 1917 (his death), had an 'attitude towards innovations in modes of treatment' that was 'one of considerable caution', but was 'in no wise hostile to modern methods' (Obituary, 1917). According to Hare (1962), 'belief in the idea that masturbation could cause insanity declined rapidly during the years 1885 to 1900', and he cites the changes in Maudsley's *Pathology of Mind* between its 1879 and 1895 editions. Likewise Clouston, in his 1888 Presidential Address to the Medico-Psychological Associ-ation (MPA), concluded that 'Masturbation may be an element in the production of secondary dementia in some cases, but it is not a necessary or a constant cause', and Newington had trained under Clouston (Medical Super-intendent at the Royal Edinburgh Asylum from 1873 to 1908) in Edinburgh. The *Journal of Mental Science* has a cluster of references to masturbation in the late 1880s (often related to a series of papers by Spitzka on 'Masturbatic Insanity', 1887 and 1888), but only two between 1890 and 1922, both of which (1898 and 1900) were concerned with the effects on children.

Further analyses of the Ticehurst records between 1890 and 1917 might well show a concomitant fall in references to masturbation and its treatments, although a notable increase, to over a third of admissions, in the 1886–90 period when the tide of theory seems to be turning, may indicate a considerable lag between acceptable theory and clinical fashion. Un-fortunately there seems to be no parallel Case-book quantifications of the level of masturbation in Victorian asylums. Tomes (1984) describes 'filthy habits' such as masturbation being common in the 'chronic and excited wards' (p. 236) of the Pennsylvania Hospital, and Digby (1985) states that 'men had a virtual monopoly of this type of alleged cause' (p. 210) until the end of the century, but no figures are supplied in either text.

The most detailed account of masturbation, in terms of prevalence and significance, is to be found in Ellis's *Studies in the Psychology of Sex* (1st edn, 1900) under the heading 'Auto-Eroticism' (pp. 161–283). Exhaustively survey-ing the literature relating psychiatric conditions to chronic masturbation (see especially pp. 248–266), Ellis points out 'there really is no end to the list of real or supposed symptoms and results of masturbation', (p. 249) and suggested that 'we may thus dismiss the extravagant views widely held during the past century, concerning the awful results of masturbation, as due to ignorance and false tradition'. But he did insist, in the same paragraph, that neurasthenia is 'probably the most important of the compara-tively frequent results' of masturbation – 'though this also arises usually on a somewhat morbid soil'. It seems that even among the most sceptical commentators the notion of mastur-bation being related to some particular diagnosis could not be dismissed. The evidence from Ticehurst (Table 6) illustrates this tendency, since the great majority of 'self-abusers' fall into the categories of 'schizophrenia' and 'in-definite', reinforcing a sense of nosological coherence. 'Masturbational insanity' may be regarded therefore as a prototype of the de-mentia praecox category, dismissed on the basis of a false aetiology but robust in its delineation of a chronic, disinhibited form of behaviour associated with a severe, primary psychopath-ology.

VIOLENCE AND RESTRAINT

Whatever standpoint is chosen, it is clear that violent and self-destructive behaviour was a major influence on asylum management and day-to-day practice. Roughly one in four of all patients exhibited violence, yet only just over one in four of these (22·4%) were deemed 'recovered' or 'cured', so the enduring of blows, bites or scratches was not usually relieved by the likely prospect of a positive outcome. Given that Ticehurst could select an upper-class, 'genteel', clientele and discharge or transfer those deemed too difficult, it is likely to have avoided re-sponsibility for the most difficult customers. The details of those put under restraint (16 patients)

between 1861 and 1890 (Table 10) illustrate some of the relevant diagnostic and outcome features of this cohort. Again, the questionable relevance of nosological precision as an aid to management is apparent.

As regards modern diagnosis, recovery was largely confined to the manic-depressive group. But 'restraint/violence' did *not* alter length of stay within diagnostic groups. Increasing with length of stay if 'schizophrenic', more charac-teristic of the shorter-stay 'manic-depressives', it seems again to isolate these groups from each other. Such figures may also provide the reasons for the continued, and optimistic, active man-agement of violent patients who had only recently been admitted. Enduring chronic, re-lapsing violence may have been eased by the expectation of improvement at least in these acute 'manic-depressive' patients. By contrast, those with 'organic' or 'indefinite' diagnoses were more likely to exhibit violence the longer they stayed. Such a cohort, continuing to deteriorate despite "moral suasion" over many years, can only have further weakened reliance on moral therapy. Extrapolating such data to the larger public asylums must be done with caution, but it would not be unreasonable to suggest that this chronic cohort would have been no less represented.

Some of the specific details of those restrained are outlined in Table 10. These cases highlight some of the themes discussed above. The four described as 'cured' or 'recovered' had well-defined manic or major depressive illnesses. At least six (i.e. 38%) were transferred to alternative care, usually another asylum. None of the five in the 'schizophrenia' category had a good out-come. On average, this group was biased towards a younger age (33·6 years) than the overall cohort, only two patients being over 41.

Length of stay was extremely variable, 50% spending less than one year in the asylum, but only one patient remaining for more than five years. There is no indication from the notes, these data or the diagnoses – whether modern or nineteenth-century – as to why restraint was (apparently) so little used in Ticehurst in the 1870s or 1880s as compared to the 1860s. It may have been related to the 'great restraint contro-versy', as outlined by Tomes (1988). It may have been a deliberate policy to select a more tractable clientele or transfer out anyone likely to need

Table 10. *Cases in Ticehurst requiring restraint, 1860–1890*

Case no.	Date	Age*	Sex†	Length of stay (months)	Outcome‡	Contemporary diagnosis	Modern diagnosis
138	1861	40	F	2	'Too violent', Removed to Dr Thomas's; sent home 'so bad'	Mania	Schizophrenia (probable)
157	1863	38	F	48	Recovered + aftercare	Delusions	Mania
164	1863	32	M	36	Died (congestion of lungs)	General paralysis	GPI
171	1864	37	M	7	Cured	Delusions	Major depression
188	1865	26	M	9	'Rational tho' somewhat (?) exciteable'	Delusions	Mania
192	1865	23	F	4	Unimproved (Dr. G. Brook House)	Delusions	Schizophrenia (probable)
197	1865	27	F	10	Not improved, removed by her parents	Mania with hysteria	?
224	1867	30	M	48	Died	Melancholia after mania	Bipolar (manic-depressive)
231	1867	54	M	42	Not improved	Mental excitement	Bipolar (manic-depressive)
239	1868	41	F	17	Recovered	Acute mania	Mania
240	1868	39	F	> 288	(Continuing in hospital 1890)	Acute mania	Schizophrenia
252	1869	60	M	3	Recovered	Mania	Major depression
254	1869	27	M	2	Transferred to Camberwell House	Mania	Mania
293	1872	19	F	24	Transferred to Northampton Asylum	Addresses imaginary persons	Schizophrenia
482	1883	25	F	4	Discharged to 'another asylum'	Acute mania	Mania
564	1888	19	M	> 24	(Continuing in hospital 1890)	Mania	Schizophrenia

* Average age 33·6 years.   † Females 8, males 8,   ‡Recovered/cured 4.

restraining. Three of the last four patients (i.e. those put under restraint between 1869 and 1888) in Table 10 were discharged to another asylum, highlighting the unusual degree of care for the last one, H. L. (admitted June 1888). This nineteen-year-old ex-Malvern College schoolboy was violent, constantly 'attacking his man' and 'eating his faeces', 'masturbated 15 times in spite of the presence of 2 men', and tended to spit, urinate in his bed and curse everyone. Treated with the mustard pack, fed by the stomach pump, his foreskin blistered with liquor Epispasticus, and confined 'by means of a jacket with long sleeves', he represents the most difficult of management problems. He even had 'asylum ear', also known as haematoma auris, and elaborately described over five pages and with many references in Tuke's *Dictionary of Psychological Medicine* (1892, pp. 557–62). One can only assume that personal or economic factors ensured his continuing stay in Ticehurst.

Comparing this experience with other work on asylums is made difficult by the lack of quantified data. Digby (1985) reports some patients at The Retreat as 'too violent for contact to be beneficial' (p. 193) and describes the use of restraint and seclusion in several of the appended case-histories. She gives an incidence of between 3% and 7% for cases restrained (p. 81) but 'the frequency with which mechanical restraint was used declined dramatically: from 1847 to 1852 there were only 16 such cases,...and thereafter it became even rarer' (p. 82). However, it seems that 'during the 1870s and 1880s the Retreat used chloral or chloral with bromide on an extensive scale', and that there was in particular a 'marked rise' in medication 'for what Dr Baker diagnosed as "excitement"' (p. 129). Digby uses the term 'chemical restraint' – as did Scull (1979) – and it may well be that the frequent use of opiates, bromides and chloral at Ticehurst during the same period (this has not been quantified because of the difficulty in interpreting shorthand pharmacological terms, but future analysts might consider such an approach) was associated with the reduced amount of restraint discussed above. A random sample of 20 patients consecutively admitted between 1883 and 1884 confirmed only four as definitely given sedative medication, while another five received some form of physical therapy (e.g. shower bath, electricity, mustard pack, suppository), but these figures may be an underestimate, since the briefer notations of drug therapy might have been missed.

The problems of violence and restraint also permeate Tomes's monograph on the Pennsylvania Hospital (1984). 'Troublesome patients posed an unavoidable and significant problem in Kirkbride's asylum practice' (p. 236). 'Throughout the period from 1750 to 1880, families confined the insane for the same types of behaviours: violence to self or others, destructiveness and extreme troublesomeness' (p. 124). 'Preventing or containing patient violence constituted the most demanding portion of the attendants' duties' (p. 180). However, 'Kirkbride appears to have used physical restraint very sparingly and carefully' (p. 198), and only when 'after being treated with narcotics, patients continued to behave in an extremely violent, life-threatening manner' (p. 197). However, no figures are available as to the proportion of patients deemed violent, or in need of restraint, just as Hunter & MacAlpine give no detailed figures for their study of Colney Hatch (1974). The latter do report that in August 1859 the Earl of Shaftesbury visited the asylum and wrote that 'out of 1491 patients, not one was under restraint or seclusion' (p. 87), but such methods were revived, not least because of staff limitations (one attendant to 12 patients, and 'only two directing physicians' for an asylum with more than 2000 patients). The superintendent, Dr Sheppard, was apparently black-balled at the Royal College of Physicians because of measures 'not resorted to in any other of the English asylums, in several of which the patients are quite as violent, dirty and destructive in their habits as the worst at Colney Hatch' (p. 86). They also report the problems caused to the asylum by 'criminal lunatics', and 'patients discharged "uncured" from other hospitals like Bethlem and St Luke's which, unlike country asylums, could afford to be selective because they were outside the service' (p. 185). Apparently, 'fractures due to fits, faints, falls, fights and even football ran at about 0·5–1% of inmates per annum', but 'injury from assault was in fact rare, contrary to the public image of asylums' (p. 187).

Violence as a significant factor in public asylum life has also been detailed by Finnane (1981) in his study of Irish asylums. 'Everyday life in the asylum was centred on the continual struggle to wrest some order out of the chaos which surrounded doctors and attendants... restlessness and agitation could easily be translated into violence between inmates' (p. 208). Likewise, Garton (1988), describing the Australian asylums, emphasized both the violence attending admission and the 'large number of complaints concerning the violence of attendants and nurses' (p. 175). To what extent this was due to staffing problems is uncertain, but the increasing need for restraint in the post-war years was apparently related to manpower shortages. According to Dwyer (1987), 'Violent patients posed a particularly troublesome challenge' at Utica and Willard Asylums in New York, and 'their casebook records overflow with stories of patients attacking one another' (p. 138). Finally, a recent study of The Retreat (Renvoize & Beveridge, 1989) also comments that 'assaults by patients on staff or fellow patients' were 'surprisingly common'.

Overall, it is difficult to be certain where Ticehurst should be placed in any hierarchy of in-patient violence. Its provision of care using large numbers of attendants – 'the large staff employed at Ticehurst was a great blessing, and all of them (i.e. asylum doctors) wished they could afford it' – enabled it to cope with some extremely disturbed patients. The ability to discharge or transfer was also used, particularly in the 1870s and 1880s (see Table 10). While taking a rich clientele, highly selected from those whom not even expensive home-care could deal with, and therefore likely to be most disturbed, it could select patients deemed appropriate for the quality of the surroundings and the required tone of gentility. Whether its patients were therefore more violent than those of the average pauper asylum must remain as yet uncertain, although this does seem inherently unlikely. But the importance of such behaviour in moulding a philosophy of care, and a diagnostic or prognostic system, cannot be ignored.

SUICIDE, 'ATTEMPTED' SUICIDE AND SUICIDAL RISK

The three definite cases of suicide reported from the Casenotes provide little material for a detail analysis. Their gender – all were male – ages and diagnoses would put them into a category of risk accepted today. The more standardized admission notes for the later 1870s, and the 1880s, include a clear requirement to state whether a patient is 'suicidal', 'epileptic' or 'dangerous'. Using these data, supplemented by details from the certificates when no clear category was indicated, it was possible to draw up Tables 8A and 8B giving the details of 100 randomly selected patients deemed at risk of suicide. The numbers are small, but 31% of admissions in this period (1876–81) points to the significance of suicidal behaviour as a precipitant for admission. To lose, apparently, only three patients in 45 years, out of over 600 admissions, when nearly one-third were brought in because of that risk, reinforces the themes apparent in the previous section. Staff, both attendants and other domestics, had to be numerous, well trained and organized. At Colney Hatch, in 1888, after two suicides in that year, a system of Suicidal Caution Cards was instituted, but it seems that one or two suicides regularly occurred per annum (Hunter & MacAlpine, 1974, pp. 188–190).

Comparative data on the prevalence of attempted suicide and suicide in relation to asylum admission and care is not difficult to come by. Parry-Jones (1972) reported only two deaths from suicide between 1828 and 1856 at Hook Norton and Witney, out of 745 patients (p. 216). However, only 28 of these admissions were officially described as 'suicidal' prior to admission (with another 48 deemed 'suicidal and dangerous'), not least because it was only after 1845 that such information was required on admission documents. He did report five suicides at Brislington House between 1830 and 1843, but regarded his overall figures as 'in keeping with the low recorded incidence of suicide in asylums in the mid-nineteenth century' (p. 213).

Tomes (1984) did not quote figures, but stressed the importance of suicidal behaviour in shaping the admission, management and design features of the Pennsylvania asylum. 'Suicidal attempts or intentions prompted many admissions to Kirkbride's mental hospital...let family members detect preparation for suicide, and commitment would surely follow' (p. 110). Furthermore, 'Kirkbride's attention to doors and windows also reflected his fear of suicide', such that windows, 'furniture that had no projections,

sharp corners, or other facilities for self-injury' and bathing facilities were carefully chosen (pp. 144–145). Likewise 'self-destructive cases' often involved the attendants keeping 'a twenty-four-hour watch to prevent any self-injury' (p. 180). Nevertheless suicides did occur, reinforcing the superintendent's conviction 'that the most trivial aspects of asylum discipline had to be enforced in order to prevent suicide, a "great and never-ending source of anxiety" for him' (p. 185).

There are also no figures from Digby's (1985) study of The Retreat at York. It seems that 'suicidal propensities were frequently recorded but suicides themselves were rare', and surveillance increasingly replaced restraint as the means of prevention. Anderson (1988), however, has provided a detailed review (pp. 376–417) of the role of medical men in suicide management, and useful comparative figures. She pointed out the considerable, apparent, success of asylums in caring for suicidal patients, since only 'a minute proportion of deaths in these institutions was ever caused by a suicidal act within them; 0·63% in 1867...and a miniscule 0·14% in 1911'. She quoted Savage as reporting that 20–30% of admissions to Bethlem were registered suicidal (p. 405), and Hood's *Statistics of Insanity* as 'reporting 38% of those admitted had meditated or attempted suicide' (p. 417). But while these figures accord with the Ticehurst findings, she stressed the likely exaggeration of suicidal tendencies in certification procedures, and the agreement of contemporary alienists (e.g. Bucknill, Savage) that this was occurring. She also pointed out the likelihood of good recovery among such patients (p. 406), not least because of the prevalence of melancholia as a diagnosis. Thus 'between 1879 and 1888 half the asylum patients who were admitted with suicidal propensities were classified as suffering from melancholia, as against only 14% of the other patients admitted', and melancholia was 'the most curable of all varieties of insanity'. Interestingly, Ticehurst's 'suicidal' cohort has 20 (out of 31) deemed melancholic (i.e. 64·5%), although only 76 out of the whole cohort (i.e. 12·6%) were labelled primarily as such, proportions that differ even more than Anderson's general figures. Such evidence supports a notion of selective admission by the Newingtons, in choosing 'manic-depressive' patients whose likely recovery could be assured given the care that their asylum (large numbers of attendants, good resources, close attention to daily events) provided.

We do in fact have available Hayes Newington's attitude to the management of suicidal patients, in a paper read to the MPA Quarterly Meeting on 9 November 1886, concerning the 'Tests of Fitness for Discharge from Asylums' (Newington, 1887). Concentrating on suicide, he suggested 'it is the loss of self-control which dominates the question of suicide, and therefore to the loss or recovery of it must we pay the chief attention'. Admitting that 'in the earlier days of my acquaintance with insanity, suicide was to me a dread possibility which overshadowed all other considerations' he proposed certain risk factors (e.g. pain, illness) and 'checks' (e.g. physical fear of death) that needed to be taken into account. Mentioning advanced dementia, alcohol, 'stomach melancholia' and insomnia as significant conditions, he ended with a reasonably confident assertion of being able to ask a patient directly and analyse the reply confidently.

The Ticehurst figures also accord, in terms of diagnosis and outcome, with those reported by Anderson from 'brief sampling' of Colney Hatch Asylum's 'Registers and Casebooks' (p. 407). She suggested that perhaps more than half of the suicidal melancholics admitted may have been discharged 'relieved' or 'well' within 18 months, and quoted Drs Rayner and Clouston as reporting similar figures. While the meaning of terms such as 'relieved' and 'recovered' cannot be assumed to validate the fact of a cure, the 21 (out of 31) suicidal cases in the Ticehurst cohort deemed 'relieved/improved/cured' match Anderson's findings. It is also clear from Tables 8A and 8B that 'melancholia' (15 out of 20 cases) has a good outcome, as does the RDC diagnosis of major (or minor) depression. The only difference lies in the nearly equal proportion of each sex in the Ticehurst cohort, as compared with Anderson's description of 'the typical asylum patient with suicidal propensity' as 'a middle-aged woman suffering from melancholia' (p. 407). This is probably due to the Newingtons' admission policy of having roughly 50:50 of each gender.

In overall terms, Ticehurst's management of suicidal patients reflected Anderson's general assertion that 'in practical terms it cannot be reckoned a failure' (p. 417). The relationship between presentation, diagnosis, outcome and modern diagnosis confirms the role of a useful nosology in selecting 'recoverable' patients. Melancholics needed watching, feeding, exercising and diversion so that self-harm might be averted until improvement, from whatever cause, took place. In fact, given the success of such cases, it may well be that attributing suicidal ideation to a prospective patient was a method of persuading reluctant relatives (several of whom insisted on remaining anonymous when first applying to Ticehurst) to accept asylum treatment or, conversely, a means whereby desperate families could persuade ambivalent physicians to transfer clinical responsibility to an asylum doctor. Such nuances can never be clarified, but the use of the term 'suicidal' clearly became pivotal in the business of certification and admission.

SPECIFIC PSYCHOPATHOLOGIES, ALCOHOL AND 'UNUSUAL' DIAGNOSES

In addition to behavioural data, the Casebooks provide a rich collection of symptoms and syndromes that have been formalized into specific entities in modern psychiatry. Some have become part of the criteria for diagnosing psychotic illness, and have been used as the key to translating the Ticehurst material into RDC diagnoses. 'Flight of ideas' and 'thought broadcast' were the most accessible in this respect, and the parallels between modern definitions and nineteenth-century usage have been outlined. The process whereby such symptoms moved from casual description to diagnostic import awaits its historian, although textbooks of the time can be shown to include versions of these criteria in their general portrayal of various states of insanity.

(i) Flight of ideas

In 1858 Bucknill & Tuke (p. 297) wrote that (in acute mania) 'the attention slips from object to object with choreic rapidity and abruptness... but, in many instances, not falsifying the judgement'. Clouston (1904, p. 160) described 'a rapid and uncontrolled passing of the ideas through the mind... a tendency to constant talking whether anyone is present or not; passing from one thing to another and soon becoming incoherence of speech', in a chapter on 'States of Mental Exaltation'. Both these texts are the most likely candidates for providing contemporary influences, being British and much reissued. Clouston's *Clinical Lectures on Mental Diseases* enlarged to a sixth edition, almost wholly by the accumulation of extra cases to reinforce his ideas. As stated earlier, Hayes Newington's training under Clouston in Edinburgh provides another obvious link.

The notion of 'Flight of ideas' was, however, widely described by the continental writers (e.g. Esquirol, Feuchtersleben, Griesinger and Kraepelin) as well as in the more practical English tradition. As the century proceeds the notion achieved increasing acceptance as diagnostic of acute mental illness, and in particular became associated by Kraepelin with recoverable, manic-depressive illness. Thus, Esquirol (1845) wrote in his chapter on 'The Symptoms of Insanity', 'the impressions are so fugitive and numerous, the ideas so abundant, that the maniac cannot fix his attention sufficiently upon each object and idea' (p. 29). In a later section, on mania, he expanded the idea that 'language... discloses the disturbance which exists in the understanding of the maniac. As thoughts present themselves in a crowd to his mind... so words and phrases escape his lips with no coherency or order, and with an extreme volubility,... they pass with the greatest rapidity from the most obliging expression to threats and abuse'. Even Feuchtersleben, in his *Principles of Medical Psychology* (1847), a work aimed at theory and philosophical analysis, in one of his few clinical asides asked 'Is giddiness from elevated position anything save the rapid flight of ideas produced by the struggle with such feelings?' (p. 298). Later he also suggested that 'occupation is here the chief physical remedy, in order to arrest the vague flight of ideas' (p. 344).

More formally, Griesinger (1867 translation of 2nd German edition, 1861) described a 'too rapid succession of the ideas' (p. 66) among the 'Elementary Disorders of Mental Disease', but elaborated this carefully in a later chapter on 'States of Mental Exaltation'. 'The first and most important change which the intellect undergoes in mania consists of an irritability and quantitative exaltation analogous to that of the disposition and the will – in a more rapid flow of ideas... there results a restless and constant succession of isolated ideas which have no intimate relation with each other, being merely connected by accidental external incidents' (p. 283). He later added a more human touch to this rather formal analysis when quoting a patients as saying 'It is actually terrible when the thoughts so run into one another in one's head' (p. 286).

By the time of Kraepelin, though, it seems that the phrase 'flight of ideas' had become established. Thus, Defendorf's (1902) translation of the 6th edition of the *Lehrbuch der Psychiatrie* has 'the speed of the maniac presents the *characteristic* flight of ideas,' (p. 198), while Johnstone's (1912) translation of the lectures has: 'in the province of the course of ideas, there arises that phenomenon which we are accustomed to call "flight of ideas"...As the idea of a goal is wanting which gives its fixed direction to healthy thought and at once arrests all side issues, the train of thought is perpetually driven out of its course, while incidental and non-essential ideas, often only awakened through habit of speed or similarity of sound, intrude everywhere...The ideas are fleeting, and soon fade again before they have actually attained clearness' (p. 64 – chapter VII on 'Maniacal Excitement'). In Defendorf the notion was also expanded (p. 292) when discussing 'hypomania'. He wrote that 'they (hypomaniacs) shift abruptly from one subject to another, and are quite unable to bring a thought to a logical conclusion... there is a striking lack of coherence in the train of thought. The patients are unable to arrange logically a series of ideas without abrupt transitions from one subject to another'. Proceeding on to describe the cardinal symptoms of mania, in bold type, he then needed only to write of 'great psychomotor restlessness with a pronounced flight of ideas'.

Similar themes of an irresistibly increased speed of thought, linking ideas randomly, following no goal-directed path, can be found throughout the English psychiatric literature of the nineteenth century. Even John Conolly (1830) in his rather diverse 'indications of Insanity' mentioned 'those [cases] in which the fancy leads the attention captive, and carries it from one idea to another without the power of resistance' (p. 346). He also quoted a Haslam case, for whom 'all the objects around... become interwoven with his narrative, and lead him from subject to subject with irresistible rapidity'. Winslow (1866) similarly wrote, 'The rapidity, as well as the loss of, volitional power over certain trains of thought, are significant and characteristic symptoms' (p. 66). Neither, however, placed the symptom clearly into a nosological framework, unlike Henry Maudsley (1895), who described ideas in acute 'mania' as 'rapid, incomplete and incoherent, the currents of them being interrupted before they are finished, and crossed at random by other ideas which in turn do not get finished' (p. 241). Several pages earlier (p. 236), in a specific description of 'Insanity with Excitement-Mania', he mentioned ideas that 'rise instantly, flow swiftly, and strike more easy and varied associations;... while the transient chance-formings of new track-junctions give rise sometimes to novel turns of thought, puns of speech...'. The later Victorian textbook writers continued such themes in some detail. Bevan Lewis (1890) discussed 'the tumultuous career of ideas...a superficial coherence may be observed which enables the patient to hold rapid converse' (p. 165), and later 'a weakening of that systematic process which renders intelligent and rational thought possible; a cohesion of ideas still is apparent but it is that of the trivial associations chiefly...the seriality of thought becomes impossible' (p. 169). Savage (1891) detailed 'the thoughts following rapidly, apparently unconnectedly, but connected...with impressions from without' (p. 115). In particular, 'In mania one is able to trace the way in which ideas and words are linked together in the mind', even though 'the condition of rapid verbal association' is associated with 'punning and verse-making' (p. 107), and 'stimulated by sense impressions without any intermediate thought-action' (p. 109). Mercier, in his very practical textbook (1902), written to 'avoid discursiveness', included a chapter on 'Acute Insanity'. In one form, apparently, the patient 'talks with rapid fluency and disconnectedly; he utters sometimes a stream of words in which each suggests the next by sound or meaning', and Mercier offered an example of such speech ('open the window, give me a glass, drink your brandy, isn't he handy? what a dandy! fine feathers make fine birds', etc.). All of these descriptions are closely followed in modern textbooks, as for example Fish's *Psychopath-*

ology (1974): '...where thoughts follow each other rapidly there is no general direction of thinking and the connexions between successive thoughts appear to be due to chance factors which, however, can usually be understood' (p. 35).

(ii) Thought broadcast

Established now as a 'first-rank' symptom of schizophrenia (Mellor, 1970), this particular form of psychotic experience hovers around a number of clinical descriptions. Patients may describe others as knowing what they (the patients) are thinking, or vice versa. A sense of one's thoughts being alien, influenced, withdrawn, inserted or controlled often intrudes on the picture. It may be argued whether it is a form of thought disorder, a delusion, or a passivity experience (see below), or even 'as the result of the breakdown of ego boundaries' (Fish, 1974, p. 81). By contrast with the increasingly standardized descriptions of 'flight of ideas' outlined above, it is much more difficult to establish a clear acceptance of this symptom in European or British texts. Just as it is recorded in the Ticehurst notes without diagnostic adumbration, so one can discover it in varying categories in the literature.

Bucknill & Tuke (1858) did not seem to mention it at all. They described a 'loss of voluntary control over the thoughts' (p. 124) as part of the second stage of dementia, and quoted Esquirol on 'persons losing their personal identity' (p. 135) in their discussion of 'false notions or conceptions' in a section on 'Delusional Insanity'. By contrast, Clouston (1904) was much more specific in a chapter on 'Monomania of Persecution, Suspicion and Unseen Agency'. He wrote of patients who 'believe that they are electrified, that they are mesmerised...that persons read their thoughts, or have power over them to act on their thoughts' (p. 259). He went on to state: 'that persons read their thoughts and influence their thoughts are very current delusions' (p. 262).

The variability in the British literature is especially perplexing given that Haslam's *Illustrations of Madness* (1810) provides possibly the richest and most colourful descriptions of thought-broadcast ever recorded. Terms like 'brain-sayings' (p. 38) ('a sympathetic communication of thought...not hearing but...a silent conveyance of intelligence'), 'kiteing' ('magnetic impregnations' that 'contrive to lift into the brain some particular idea') (p. 31) and 'thought-making' (p. 34 – 'sucking out the brain of the person assailed, to extract his existing sentiments') are hard to forget and perfectly specific. Yet there is nothing along these lines in Conolly (1830) – who quoted Haslam on other symptoms – apart from a hesitant description (pp. 343–344) of a man who 'had lost the power of directing his attention steadily to any subject'. Winslow (1866) mentioned in passing (ch. IV, 'Confessions of Patients after Recovery from Insanity', p. 66) a patient who 'thought everybody on earth knew my thoughts' but made no diagnostic comment. Maudsley (1895) suggested that 'it is a different thing when the person believes that his persecutors persistently tap this thoughts...' (p. 306) so as to emphasize the significance of certain symptoms of 'Insane Deformities of Mind'. Subsequently describing a list of symptoms of those whose 'mental degeneration increases gradually into dementia' (p. 405), he wrote that 'they ascribe in like manner to telepathic, telephonic, or other occult agency... their inability to control their wandering thoughts'... 'by which their true thoughts are obstructed, tapped, turned on to wrong lines...' (p. 406).

Interestingly, Bevan Lewis (1890) included a 'very special form of delusion' in a chapter on 'Alcoholic Insanity'. 'The faculty of thought and speed become impaired... as the victim believes, by the direct operation of a power which has gained access to his brain; which rules his thoughts and dictates its very utterances... where no sensory hallucination has been experienced' (p. 319). This seems more a version of thought insertion, but Lewis's contemporary, Savage (1890), included a more detailed description of 'Thought-Reading' in a chapter on 'Delusional Insanity' (p. 241). 'There are always patients whose chief complaint is that persons know their thoughts or know more about them than they ought... such patients may say they have "loud thoughts"'. He gave an example of a man who 'had committed assaults upon people for no other reason than that they knew too much about him', and who climbed a hillock on Hampstead Heath each morning 'to keep a look out that no one was observing him or taking his thoughts away from him'. Mercier (1902),

however, regarded these symptoms as part of 'Paranoia'. 'It is more common for the mysterious influence to be exerted upon the mind. Other people read their thoughts, or think their thoughts, or put thoughts into their minds or deprive them of the power of thinking....'

Going back into the continental literature, it is very difficult to find any clear examples in Esquirol (1845) or Feuchtersleben (1847). But Griesinger (1867) did point to the difficulty of understanding these symptoms in his chapter on 'Elementary Disorders in Mental Disease'. He stated, 'we cannot form any clear conception of what is meant when we hear insane persons complain that their thoughts are entirely made for them by others, or that they are abstracted from them' (p. 62). He later quoted a case of 'Chronic Mania with Delusions and Hallucinations of Hearing' as asking 'How does it happen that you heard my thoughts?' (p. 335). Kraepelin (Defendorf, 1902) had no compunction in placing them under 'Dementia Praecox – Paranoid Form', as a well known and common symptom. 'Others complain that their minds are influenced, their thoughts are gone, they have no control over their thoughts... they attribute the origin of such thoughts to others which are forced upon them in spite of themselves' (pp. 193–194). In Johnstone's 1912 translation of the 'Lectures' a Dementia Praecox patient is described as having his thoughts 'construed' – 'what I have thought, the others have said' (p. 166). But the author's dictum that one should 'never rely too much, in making a diagnosis, on the presence or absence of any one symptom', and 'always keep the general picture' before one's eyes seems particularly relevant with this type of symptom. Unlike 'flight of ideas' it lacked a diagnostic or prognostic weight. Its haphazard occurrence in the Ticehurst notes provides a nice link with current nosology, and accords with the confusion as to its contemporary diagnostic relevance.

(iii) Unusual diagnoses

The presence of Capgras delusions and Cotard's syndrome (see Table 11 for case details), erotomania and rarer forms of anorexia and alcohol-induced states (e.g. Korsakoff's psychosis) further reinforces the recognizability and severity of psychopathology encountered in Ticehurst. It is unnecessary to discuss these

Table 11. *Patients at Ticehurst presenting with Capgras or Cotard's syndrome (1850–1890)*

Capgras (N = 16)						Cotard's (N = 14)					
Case no.	Age	Sex	V/R*	RDC diagnosis†	Outcome	Case no.	Age	Sex	V/R*	RDC diagnosis†	Outcome
108	37	F	V+R	M-D	Restored	129	40	M	—	M-D	Died (Suicide)
112	23	M	V	M-D	Died	195	35	M	—	Organic (GPI)	Died
143	53	M	—	S	Not improved	219	70	M	—	M-D	Died
208	52	F	—	M-D	Recovered	242	75	F	—	M-D	Died
250	38	F	—	S	Recovered	262	61	M	—	M-D	Died
281	38	F	—	M-D	Not improved	268	60	M	—	M-D	Cured
297	56	M	—	S	Not relieved	287	62	M	V	M-D	Relieved
303	26	F	—	S	Discharged	296	42	M	—	M-D	Died
355	48	F	V	S	—	307	55	M	V	M-D	Died
331	33	F	—	M-D	Relieved	315	62	M	—	M-D	Not improved
335	68	M	—	Organic	Died	339	39	M	V	Organic (GPI)	Died
434	24	F	V	S	Unimproved	427	53	F	V	M-D	Relieved
442	37	F	—	S	Relieved	473	60	F	—	M-D	Relieved
482	25	F	V+R	M-D	Discharged	485	72	F	—	Organic (dementia)	Died
511	25	M	—	S	—						
574	30	F	V	?	—						

* Violence/restraint.   † M-D, manic depressive; S, schizophrenic; ?, uncertain.

presentations in detail, since they are conditions whose nosological status remains uncertain.

(a) Capgras syndrome

The Capgras delusion has provoked a considerable literature in recent years, not least because of its mythical and historic interest (*Lancet*, 1986). But the association with significant organic pathology has also led to speculation that it may provide the first direct link between a specific cerebral lesion and a specific psychopathology.

The nineteenth-century literature does contain hints as to its occurrence, as in Winslow's (1866) statement about a female patient who 'at times had serious doubts as to her personal identity' (p. 60). Griesinger (1867) also mentioned 'loss of personal identity' (p. 335), but misidentification of someone else is much more apparent in the later, turn-of-the-century literature. Thus, Maudsley (1895) intoned against 'all sorts of false perceptions; familiar faces seem as strange faces, whence utmost distrust of them' (p. 246), which is confusing since it is not specific enough and stresses misperception rather than false belief. Savage (1891), however, delighted in telling of a 'most extraordinary series of delusions', in a case illustrating 'Delusional Insanity'

(p. 265). He described a patient whose wife left the room temporarily during a domestic card game but, 'although he remained just as he had been...another woman, resembling her in every outward particular, took her place, assuming her seat at the card table and accompanying him to bed'. The patient went on to believe that 'Roman Catholics' were 'substituting duplicates' for his wife and children (p. 266). This is very specific, and such multiple misidentifications were also mentioned by Clouston (1904), particularly in quoting a patient's letter (e.g. 'Old Captain G....is here; he calls himself Dr. S. but I don't mind that') in a chapter on 'Fixed and Limited Delusion (Monomania, Mono-Psychosis, Paranoia' (p. 249).

The Ticehurst cohort of Capgras patients fits into this ill-defined nosology in that they tend to have a poor outcome, related to persisting psychotic illness. Comparison with the most extensive modern cohort (Berson, 1983), nearly 20% of whom had clear 'organic' illness, while less than one-sixth (20 out of 133) had 'manic-depressive' diagnoses, shows a considerable bias, however, towards the latter category (37·5%) in the Ticehurst group. The numbers are small, but this difference may once more indicate the greater severity of manic-depressive illness (regarded by many modern psychiatrists as essentially organic in origin, although the pathology has yet to be established) in Victorian times. As Hare (1981) has pointed out, the nineteenth-century psychiatric textbook descriptions 'of typical cases of acute mania' are 'not much like the kind of psychiatric diseases we see today'. He noted also the incidence of 'epileptic insanity' (5–10% of admissions), GPI (some 20% of admissions) and 'alcoholic insanity' (about 5% of admissions), and the higher contemporary mortality rate of asylum inmates. The possibility that these more severe presentations were early forms of GPI, or secondary to obscure cerebral diseases, therefore remains strong. By contrast the proportion deemed 'schizophrenic' at Ticehurst (nine out of sixteen, including one 'uncertain' (see Fig. 3); that is, 56·3%) compares well with Berson's figure of 77 out of 133 (i.e. 57·6%), so it is not unreasonable to equate these groups despite the lack of apparent 'organic' features noted above. (N.B. The 'uncertain' case was described as 'lost', 'irritable', 'in all kinds of attitudes' and 'full of delusions', but she lacked enough positive symptoms to fulfil strict research criteria for what appears clinically a very schizophrenia-like disorder.)

(b) Cotard's syndrome

The fourteen cases in the notes accord closely with those outlined in Jules Cotard's 1882 paper 'Du délire des négations' (Hirsch & Shepherd, 1974, pp. 354–373), wherein he described 'a particular type of delusional formation which seems to me to develop in a considerable number of melancholic patients'. He stressed the 'habitually negativistic tendencies exhibited by these patients', characterized by anxiety, suicidal ideas, and food refusal (six out of fourteen Ticehurst patients had to be force-fed by the stomach tube). He also presented case-histories in three categories, namely nihilistic delusions 'in their simplest form', as 'symptomatic of GPI', and 'in association with delusions of persecution'. This is matched by the two (possibly three – one dementia case is of uncertain origin) cases of GPI in the Ticehurst cohort, and the presence of some persecutory ideas amid the guilt and negativism of the patients' delusions. Thus, G.J. (admitted December 1871) presented with certificates recording his delusions about people who 'conspired to drug him', and the Revd W.T. (admitted August 1873) complained of 'imaginary ill-treatment' and imagined he was 'under Satanic influence'. In fact, this clergyman patient went on to claim that he was 'possessed with the Devil', which reflects exactly Cotard's third category, 'wherein patients think of themselves as possessed rather than demented' (p. 364). Cotard himself equated it with Esquirol's heading of 'Demonomania', concluding that it 'seems to me to constitute a sort of transition between delusions of guilt and delusions of persecution'.

The condition was also regularly described in English textbooks of the period, Bevan Lewis (1890), Maudsley (1895) and Clouston (1904) giving clear accounts, and even for once agreeing as to its classification as part of 'Hypochondriacal Melancholia'. Bevan Lewis described 'delusive conceptions of the absence or total occlusion of the gullet' (p. 144), and patients who 'declare that they have no stomach' (p. 145). Maudsley, in similar vein, gave as an example a patient who 'imagines that his gullet is contracting or actually closed ... or that he has no stomach, or that his bowels never act, while he is all the while taking food or having it regularly forced on him in spite of his protests' (p. 231). This is very much the experience of the Ticehurst cohort, and may even have been subconsciously copied by Clouston, who described 'cases who affirm they have no stomachs nor gullets and that their bowels are not moved for years etc.' (p. 56). Clouston actually elaborated a list of the delusions of 100 melancholics (pp. 79–80), which included 'having no stomach', 'having no inside', and 'having neither stomach nor brains'.

A final point of agreement between Cotard and the Ticehurst data is the poor prognosis. According to the former, 'the patients arrive at a systematized delusional state from which recovery rarely occurs' (p. 363), although 're-covery, when it occurs, is as sudden as the onset' (p. 362). Only one patient left Ticehurst 'cured' (from the fourteen identified) and the recovery was certainly rather sudden after an admission of some thirty months. Such agreement of description amongst contemporaries, and of diagnosis across time (melancholia with hypochondriasis/delusions in the late nineteenth century, matched by major depressive disorder in the late twentieth century) indicates how much more precise is a nosology based on content rather than form. Garton (1988) related a number of cases from Australia in which 'the central feeling was that of loss of bodily sensations', patients describing 'how they felt as if they had no organs in their body' (p. 140). Noting a female preponderance, he was led to consider 'constructions of femininity', without reviewing the underlying diagnoses. While it is of interest that the Ticehurst cohort is over two-thirds male (perhaps a selection bias due to underlying GPI or even a counterbalance to the Asylum's apparent collection of manic females), the lack of diagnostic coherence points to a much more empirical approach. While avoiding the snares of labelling on the basis of delusional content, it may well have been a policy decision after 1875 to limit male 'Cotardist' admissions (the three cases after this year are all female) because of their poor prognosis. We only have the limited evidence of the 1857–73 Casebook to suggest selectivity, but it does show three times as many applications as admissions, as well as a number of 'declined' patients. Once more it is possible to suggest that the priorities of the private institutions were practical. Learned classifications, whether by English or Continental authors, helped little in the need to maintain a turnover, a cure-rate even, so as to keep one's reputation, and, perhaps, keep up staff morale. Negativistic patients, one might speculate, did not promote positive thinking.

(c) *Other diagnoses*

The small number of cases that fit categories of erotomania ('de Clérambault's syndrome'), neurological syndromes, eating disorders and puerperal illness make detailed discussion inappropriate. The textbook sources used to illustrate other forms of psychopathology similarly describe a range of cases that conform to these disorders.

Erotomania has a long history, as outlined by Baruk (Hirsch & Shepherd 1974, pp. 375–383) quoting in particular De Clérambault's 1921 paper on 'Les Psychoses Passionels'. Esquirol has a section entitled Erotomania (pp. 335–342) in which a number of cases are described, and even Feuchtersleben (1847) mentions 'the insanity of love, erotomania distinguished from

nymphomania...it fastens upon some object whose past or present possession it imagines' (pp. 280–281). Maudsley suggested that 'women are more prone than men to similar love-manias', pointing out that 'there may be nothing mad in the demeanour and conduct of such a victim of erotomania' (p. 321). Clouston (1904) briefly noted 'women of middle life with the combined delusion that certain men want to marry them, but that other people are preventing this' (p. 267). Kraepelin (in the Defendorf translation, 1902) included 'erotic cases' whenever 'the patient usually believes himself the object of admiration by some lady', such that 'numerous fantastic methods of communicating his love to her are devised' (pp. 321–322). But this is seen merely as a type of 'Paranoia', which seems an appropriate category for the single Ticehurst patient, Capt. Childe, who had such symptoms.

As for the eating disorders (anorexia nervosa and bulimia), Clouston (1904) mentioned 'the fasting girls' among 'the girls with stigmata, those who see visions of the Saviour...fall into trances' as instances of 'Hysterical Insanity' (p. 533), and the same category was used by Kraepelin (pp. 249–250) to discuss patients with 'the most varied ailments' who 'have been through the most remarkable forms of treatment'. Maudsley (1895) had a 'third variety' of adolescent insanity, 'the strange moral perversion and intellectual obliquity displayed in some cases of hysteria'. Included among them were 'those who, professing to live without food, attract the curiosity and excite the gaping wonder of the whole countryside' (p. 397), but although Gull's original description of anorexia was published during this period (Gull, 1874), it is clear that Ticehurst did not admit many cases where 'moral perversion' was a primary problem.

The diagnosis of 'moral insanity' was contentious enough, as the discussion at a BMA meeting in 1884, after a paper by Hack Tuke, amply shows (Discussion, 1885). Dr George Savage reckoned there were 'two classes of hysteria, one the Rossetti-like women, who, like the grave, seem ever hungry; and the second, women who were gross, fat, and sensual looking. There were two similar classes of morally insane...perversion at puberty...in other cases there is mathematical or musical power...

though morally insane.' Dr Yellowlees stated that 'in the individual the perversion is usually congenital', differentiated it from epilepsy, suggested that 'when the full history is known' such patients 'die from brain disease', but insisted 'they are most unwelcome inmates of an asylum'. This latter comment was echoed by Dr Wiglesworth, who felt they were 'the curse of every asylum to which they are sent', while Dr Conolly Norman raised the problem 'that the insane may simulate insanity'. Dr Tuke considered that 'clinical facts established the existence of the morbid mental condition' but agreed that 'volitional power' being the mental function that was lost, it was difficult to include this as legal evidence of insanity.

There is one Ticehurst case (H. B.) representative of this condition, and the absence of others like him is striking but significant. As Hayes Newington stated at an MPA meeting in July 1886, 'it was principally the "moral insanity" cases which made the most noise from the patients point of view, and they were just the people in asylums whose opinions should be considered the least' (*Journal of Mental Science*, **32**, 301). H.B.'s case was definitely 'congenital' according to Newington's notes, which were continually infused with considerable undertones of distaste. It seems that the structural regime of Ticehurst, with its walks, feeding methods and medical approach was inappropriate for such patients, and in general they were carefully excluded. It seems inappropriate therefore to regard the Newington's diagnostic and prognostic skills as rudimentary (cf. MacKenzie, 1985, p. 169). They had developed a system for managing acute and chronic behaviour disturbance secondary to psychotic illness. That was their business and their expertise.

The numbers of patients with obvious illness, already discussed, would have anyway justified their medical and nursing approach. If we consider also the impact of the odd neurological states (e.g. stupor, Korsakoff's psychosis) and puerperal illnesses, these would have reinforced an organic model of mental illness as brain disease. While GPI provided the most glaring link between psychotic symptoms, such as delusions and hallucinations, and physical signs (e.g. tremor, gait disturbance, fits), the complications induced by alcohol abuse were well known among contemporaries. Bevan Lewis (1890) devoted a large section (pp. 288–333) to 'Alcoholic Insanity' and Mercier (1902) included 'Insanity from Alcohol' (pp. 158–164) in a long chapter that contained sections on stupor and puerperal insanity. In particular he noted the prominence of a memory disorder wherein 'the current events of daily life are swept out of the memory as soon as they have happened', often accompanied by a 'peculiar delusion of memory' in which 'the patient remembers vividly and in detail events which have never occurred at all'.

Yet while an organicist, and thus medical, diagnosis was indicated in some patients, it is clear that outside the 1860s the Newingtons seem to have avoided such admissions. Not only was it difficult to enforce abstention in a large institution using brandy, champagne and porter as part of the usual 'dietary', but the relapse of several delirium tremens cases cannot have been welcome. Furthermore these cases, though obviously 'organic' if delirious or hallucinatory or neurologically impaired, could also be seen as morally perverse by their weakness in relapsing back into 'habits of intemperance'. The late Victorians' dilemma in coping with habitual drunkards, whether morally or legally, is outlined by MacLeod (1967), who highlights the difficulties of definition and disagreements as to the cause of alcoholism. While the reforming group were successful in defining it as a 'nervous disease' rather than a 'moral vice', the available 'cures' were difficult to enforce in a society jealous of individual liberty. Nevertheless 'an overestimation of the value of asylum treatment' (Brown, 1985) led to the establishment of a number of specialist inebriate asylums. As with other aspects of this diagnostic analysis, the discarding of its alcoholic clientele can be seen as typical of Ticehurst's self-limiting role. The expanding definitions of mental disorder associated with professional developments, the enlarging asylum population, and categories of neurasthenia and other neurotic states, were perhaps too much for one relatively small institution. The bluff and energetic Hayes Newington may have written the key description of Mania à Potu (Newington, 1874) in his youth, but at Ticehurst he seems to have concentrated on providing care for mainline 'true' psychosis, untrammelled by the morally doubtful problems of personality or dependency. Such an approach is illustrated in particular by the treatments and language of notation used in the asylum, as will be outlined in the next section.

(iv) Other therapies

Little has been written as yet of the details of the psychological approaches applied to Ticehurst, not least because it is difficult to get a clear outline of their nature. The use of a wide range of occupations and amusements is well documented, with routine notes describing walks, picnic, entertainments, lectures by Mr Grossmith, drives, hunting and cricket. A common lament of private asylum owners was the difficulty of getting their patients to do anything, since many simple occupations were regarded as below the dignity of a gentleman or lady. Thus, Dr Eastwood, (1863) recorded that 'the means of occupation for private patients is one of the most difficult things the physician has to deal with'. He went on, 'it is almost impossible to find actual employment for gentlemen...a few will spend some of their time in gardening and farm work, but their position prevents them from doing more than this'. It was easier with female patients 'because the needle is a resource for every class'.

The Newingtons (*Medical Superintendents*, 1901) echoed such sentiments, stating that 'we find it impossible to induce the class we have to deal with to undertake anything in the way of manual labour against their will', explaining how 'at one time we went to much expense in laying out a garden and building a large greenhouse for the special purpose of interesting the patients in their own work, but we soon found it a hopeless task trying to get them to do anything or take any interest whatever'. They mentioned 'a pack of foot-harriers...but here again it is most difficult to create any enthusiasm for it'. Amusements like 'theatrical and other entertainments, besides weekly dances during the colder months', were apparently enjoyed. Finally, 'a fair number take a more or less perfunctory interest in cricket and other games, and some few have a very decided liking for bicycle polo. This latter is a really valuable agent, as it needs such skill and direct attention to the game that their mental idiosyncrasies have little scope for action for the time being.' Such 'therapeutic virtues' were seen in other establishments also, even the public asylums.

Thus 'the game of Cricket afforded muc enjoyment and led to the recovery of som patients' at Colney Hatch in 1857 (Hunter & MacAlpine, 1974, p. 75).

Yet the underlying ethos of alienists of th time made such difficulties a cause for seriou self-doubt. In their outline of Moral Treatmen (1858), adumbrated over several editions, Buck nill & Tuke portrayed the physician as the key t successful therapy. He must have 'a firm wil the faculty of self-control, a sympathizin distress at moral pain, a strong desire to remov it' (p. 489). One must 'place the patient in a ne\ entourage of circumstances' and 'furnish inter esting and wholesome objects of thought', fo 'useful occupation is far superior to any form c amusement' (p. 493). It was felt that 'a firr steady contradiction to the truth of patient delusions' will, 'by stimulating the exercise c healthy thought', lead to 'new trains of ideas becoming 'the habit of the mind' (pp. 494–495 The authors acknowledged that 'this mode c treatment of the higher classes of society is mor difficult than that of the poor', because 'i addition to their resistance to authority they ar inapt and averse to laborious pursuits' (p. 498 Suggestions as to 'scientific gardening – sport of every kind' and 'accomplishments, paintin and music' were made, but in the end 'the mor pharmacopoeia of the physician is in his hea and in his heart' (quoting Dr Leuret, p. 501). A Clouston put it (1887, p. 491), psychiatrists wer 'priests of the body and teachers of the truths c medico-psychology' (Ray, 1981).

Burdened by such a task, what were th physicians of Ticehurst to do? Surrounded b wealthy lunatics displaying 'extraordinary atti tudes', 'vegetative', 'torpid' and 'languid random irruptions of masturbation, violenc and verbal abuse, how were they to engage i the moral task? We have the somewhat blu description (Appendix) of Hayes Newingto trying to dissuade a paranoid patient out of hi delusions, but was it successful? According t the physician, 'since then he has been quit different, cheerful, and ready to talk or d anything'. Mr P., the patient, was apparently n longer heeding his 'aural hallucinations', n longer their 'victim and slave'. While having hi 'turns', these were 'amenable to moral treat ment', and the patient was discharged to singl care with a medical man, 'relieved'. But as note earlier, this outcome category was something of a euphemism. Bowels may have been purged, flesh put on, symptoms reduced in intensity, but the patient had not been 'cured' or 'recovered'. This very much fits the 'impaired identity model' outlined by Ray (1981), in that patients 'no longer inhabit the sick role, but a stigmatised role in which identity is always impaired. Behaviour is to be maintained by social pressure to resemble normal behaviour as closely as possible, within the limits of the condition' (p. 244).

Furthermore, although 'the very existence of an asylum system for several decades meant that a family history of insanity became more visible than before' (Ray, 1981), the private clientele at Ticehurst were perhaps much less forthcoming than pauper patients. 'With us mendacity is added in probably a greater degree to ignorance of family history than is usual in most institutions', admitted the Newingtons (*Medical Superintendents*, 1901), and furthermore 'private patients tend to come into care considerably later than is the case with paupers'. In his letter to the editors of the *Journal of Mental Science* (1885), vigorously defending private asylums from the threat of abolition, Hayes Newington pointed out that 'many of the upper classes can and do retain the services of independent specialists and get well without leaving home, or are sent away to medical men's houses'. Therefore 'what we do get are not infrequently the residue of unsuccessful treatment elsewhere', since 'in the case of the wealthy it is well known that an asylum is generally the last thing thought of'. Despite 'our material' being 'more unpromising', he quoted a lower relapse rate (1:10 as opposed to about 1:7 for public asylums) and an 'average time of residence' which was 'about two-thirds of that in either a county asylum or hospital'. However, problems also arose at the other end of the admission. It seems that 'as a rule the greater the riches of a patient the greater is the tendency for the friends to remove him for trial under other circumstances, if reasonable prospect of recovery does not show itself'.

The dilemmas for the Ticehurst physicians were therefore much more practical than might be suggested in certain modern analyses. Psychiatry's 'much-vaunted special competence in the "moral treatment" of the insane' (Clark, 1983) or the dualist contradictions of moral/physical aetiology (cf. Ray, 1981, pp. 244; Foucault, 1967) do not achieve primacy as a subtext in these Casenotes. Rather one sees the 'tensions between custodial and curative roles' (Ray, 1981) obscured by random admission demands, variable exit procedures and a limited diagnostic schema. Central to moral treatment was employment, according to John Conolly (1856), yet work was by definition excluded from the 'normal' façade of genteel country-house activity. A similar situation seems to have pertained at The Retreat, as outlined by Digby (1984). 'An all-pervasive change in ethos accompanied' the development of 'outdoor facilities for sport' and 'more sophisticated' recreations. In fact, 'moral treatment was no longer a coherent philosophy of living but increasingly became trivialized into a recreational programme... a daily timetable that featured varied amusements replaced a routine that gave each ordered part of the day a moral purpose'. Even the simple management style outlined by Maudsley (1895) – 'exact account should be taken of the individual character, and the circumstances of attendance and treatment be adapted accordingly' (p. 561) – was perhaps difficult to achieve. Categories overlapped, symptoms and signs predicted variable outcomes, moral suasion and example had limited impacts, and a residual population of masturbatory, gesticulating, hallucinatory patients provided a backdrop to the most energetic of treatment regimes. It is no wonder that a modern Newington, recalling his experience as a child visiting the asylum, described it as a place he hated visiting and had largely avoided ever since (personal communication).

PHYSICAL TREATMENTS

If one considers treatment methods as outlined in contemporary textbooks, it is clear that the approach at Ticehurst conformed to accepted practices, combining a judicious mixture of the traditional and the modern. Bucknill & Tuke (1858, 1874) discussed treatment in terms of 'Hygienic', 'Moral' and 'Medicinal' approaches, although the sixteen years separating the first and third editions of their *Manual of Psychological Medicine* saw a significant expansion of the whole section on treatment (from 52 pages to 133 in fact). Admitting that 'these domains of medicine...are by no means so distinct', they outlined a regimen of nutritious foods, tonics, purgatives, stimulants, cold lotions, warm bathing and 'muscular exercise in the open air'. The choice of an appropriate form of asylum and a range of medications (tartrate of antimony, calomel, opium, purgatives, etc.) accompany a detailed account of 'Moral treatment'. They pointed out that 'no term has of late years been more profusely and empirically employed and none has been less understood' (1858, p. 486). Certain features of the Ticehurst approach accord with some of their principles, although the physicalist therapies outlined by such as Maudsley (1895) and Clouston (1904) (neither of whom separately discussed 'moral treatment') were increasingly dominant.

(i) Feeding instruments

There seems little doubt that the Newington family had an expertise in feeding procedures, stemming perhaps from Charles Newington (1781–1852), author of an 1826 paper in the *Lancet* on 'an Instrument for Administering Food'. In addition, Theodore Newington (1851–1930), when assistant medical officer at Bethlem, devised an instrument for 'Feeding by the Nose' (1879), while his cousin Hayes Newington (1877) had discussed 'Nutrient enemata' in a case-report on the management of epilepsy. It is not therefore surprising that at least 9% of the clientele at Ticehurst were fed by some artificial method, particularly since such patients often fitted the 'manic-depressive' category of curable affective illness that seems to have been selected by the Newingtons because of its better prognosis.

This technique, however, was not without its critics and its risks. In 1865 Henry Maudsley exhibited an instrument for feeding via the nostrils, on behalf of an absent MPA member. He stated that from his own experience an episode of 'near-asphyxiation' had led him since then to 'have never fed anyone except by a stomach pump'. In 1874 Bucknill & Tuke admitted that 'much diversity of practice has existed on this subject' (p. 755), but came down in preference of an oesophageal tube introduced via the mouth. 'We have never known any harm done to an insane patient by the use of the stomach-pump' they stated (p. 755), and went on to give as their 'strongest advice' that if you

'decide to feed, feed early' (p. 757). Savage (1891) was equally direct. In the treatment of acute mania he insisted that 'no feeling of sentiment should withhold the physician from feeding artificially' (p. 97). Even by the time of Clouston's 6th edn (1904) feeding remains 'one of the first considerations'. Detailing a specific form of egg custard, the author stated: 'if he [the patient] refuses absolutely it can be poured into his stomach quite early through a funnel attached to a long rubber tube, No. 12 or No. 14 catheter size (to be got from all surgical instrument makers)' (pp. 703–704).

Such a robust British approach does not seem matched by some continental authors. Reviewing *Compulsory Feeding* by Dr E. Régis in the 'French Retrospect' of April 1884 (*Journal of Mental Science* 30, 150–151), Drs McDowell and Tuke were astonished that 'the author appears to be excessively afraid of the dangers attending the passage of the oesophageal tube', insisting that 'an ordinary tube can always be passed with perfect safety if proper care be taken'. Nevertheless, in July 1885 *Journal of Mental Science* 31, 284) Dr Yellowlees reported a case of sudden death during feeding by the stomach pump, which led to a discussion as to the relative methods. 'The general opinion of the meeting was that if a patient can be as easily fed by the mouth, the oesophageal mode was preferable, but when there was much difficulty, the nasal was to be preferred'. It was also noted that 'nasal feeding has also sometimes a good moral effect on the patient', but whether this applied to the case of F.S., who refused food until she 'sees the stomach tube', is uncertain. The overlap of behavioural and 'moral effect' was exactly what Bucknill & Tuke were alluding to in their comments on 'Moral treatment'.

Notwithstanding these debates, the business of forced alimentation clearly occupied a considerable part of the day's activities at Ticehurst. The patients requiring it were psychotic and deaths did occur, but a return to normal eating habits was a common, satisfactory, outcome. When a Dr Henry Sutherland reported on 'Prognosis in Cases of Refusal of Food' (Sutherland, 1883), based on 200 patients, 18 of whom had refused food, he found he had four deaths, two 'not improved' and 12 'recovered', but expressed disappointment at the small numbers, since 'I have fed so many patients in private practice that the remembrance of their cases led me to believe I had fed a much larger number in my asylums'. From his experience he outlined seven poor prognostic features, including persistent refusal, an 'irremovable' bodily cause, persistent suicidal tendencies, loss of flesh and delayed treatment 'by drugs and proper feeding'. Hayes Newington spoke in the subsequent discussion (p. 312), suggesting that 'more incurable cases arose in the male...whereas a woman would do it with no object at all – perhaps simply hysterically – and often after a time would give in'. This may have been due to the prevalence of GPI among his male patients requiring such treatment, since females did seem to do better. But the Ticehurst figures also show a progressive improvement in the outcome of 'force-fed' patients over successive decades. Up to 1869 only three out of seventeen did well ('cured/recovered'), while during the 1880s nearly 60% (eight out of fourteen) were discharged 'recovered/relieved', including five of seven women. Newington's comment reflected a reality. The stomach tube was used on fewer admissions but perhaps more judiciously or even on a better-selected population. Certainly in 1901 the Newingtons admitted that 'it has always been a traditional practice to devote much attention to the primae viae. In 1819 our grandfather devised the first instrument for feeding patients with a tube...' but also describe the use of electricity (in hysterical patients refusing food) so as to avoid 'the use of forcible feeding' (Medical Superintendents, 1901). Such pragmatic considerations seem to have informed also their other treatment approaches.

(ii) Mustard baths/pack

This had a much less traditional role in nineteenth-century therapeutics, and the 40 cases documented show a similar pattern of declining usage during the 1880s. Nevertheless in 1901 the Newingtons could still report the effectiveness of both mustard packs and the mustard bath. 'In some cases we have found the mustard pack most useful, but this requires to be applied for some hours – in fact, it should not be removed till the patient awakes, which may be after six or seven hours.' They continued, 'we have also frequently used the mustard bath, but the action of this is not so powerful as that of the mustard pack on account of the shorter time to which the

patient can be subjected to it', and went on to describe this method (Medical Superintendents, 1901). In Tuke's *Dictionary of Psychological Medicine* (1892) there are two entries, namely 'Warm Baths medicated by Mustard' (p. 118) and on the 'Mustard Pack' (p. 123), both subsumed under the heading 'Baths', which included 15 varieties of bath treatment. The former is advocated for 'cases wherein it is desired rapidly to diminish the circulation and lower the temperature, as in acute cerebral hyperaemia'. The latter is said to have been 'only occasionally employed...so that the data as to its advantages are few'. The article mentioned the late Dr S. Newington as the first to recommend it, based on a theory of inducing sleep by abstracting blood from the head. It is said to be of value in 'cases of insanity attended by insomnia', and the high percentage of Ticehurst cases with 'mania' probably fitted into such criteria.

It is difficult to find many other references to such treatment in the standard textbooks. Bucknill & Tuke (1858 and 1874) discussed warm baths and Turkish baths, with some enthusiasm, as did Clouston (1904), but no mention of mustard is apparent. Kirkbride in Pennsylvania used 'mustard foot baths' for mania (Tomes, 1984, p. 196), but they are not reported at The Retreat (Digby, 1985). However, a good outcome was apparent in over half the cases treated at Ticehurst, particularly during the 1870s. This seems justification for the continued use of the treatment, although selection factors probably biased results. In fact, five of six recoveries in the 1880s were female, four of them suffering from 'mania'. The numbers are small but such homogeneity reinforces the view of a judiciously applied treatment based on a diagnostic and prognostic assessment. Insomnia is also a key feature of the modern criteria for manic illness, and seems to have been a target-symptom for this therapy. However, the overlap between therapy and restraint in this procedure should not be overlooked. In fact, the Newingtons had to discontinue using the mustard pack, due to 'the new rules of the Commissioners limiting the continued use of the pack to two hours', despite their belief that as a remedy it was 'in careful hands...a powerful one' (Medical Superintendents, 1901).

(iii) Electrical procedures

There is a detailed literature on treatment with electricity throughout the later nineteenth century. Bucknill & Tuke (1874, pp. 748–749) reported a series of 15 cases, nine of which responded well, and a discussion at the MPA in 1883 (*Journal of Mental Science* **29**, 318) quoted Clouston as to its efficacy, 'particularly in its stimulating influence in cases of melancholia and stupor'. A later review of three German monographs (pp. 415–424) stressed the use of 'general faradisation' in treating neurasthenia. However, Dr A. de Watteville (1885), in his *Practical Remarks on the Use of Electricity in Mental Disease*, was limited in his enthusiasm, refraining from 'committing myself to any positive statements concerning the forms of mental derangement in which electrisation [*sic*] is most likely to prove successful'. In 1892, in Tuke's *Dictionary* (pp. 426–431), electricity was said to be 'an excellent remedy', although it had to 'be applied with care and perseverance'. Its key feature was that it had 'stimulant' properties.

These factors probably explain its sparse and intermittent use at Ticehurst, even in stuporose or physically retarded patients. Since these were largely suffering from 'schizophrenic' illnesses (six out of the ten documented cases), it is not surprising that the results may have been unexceptional. It is also likely that the electrical machinery was in itself very crude. Given the prevalence (see above) of 'the electrics', 'galvinism' and 'magnetism' in the delusional passivity states of numerous patients, it may also have been felt unwise to feed their insane beliefs. The picture overall is of a preparedness to try modern forms of therapy, but of a lack of conviction after a few failures.

A recent review of the use of electricity in treatment during this period (Beveridge & Renvoize, 1988) states that, from clinical accounts, 'it was predominantly female patients who were given electric treatments, although of course there were more female than male patients in Victorian asylums'. By contrast, seven of the ten Ticehurst patients thus treated were male, which might indicate an empirical approach based on presenting symptoms (e.g. retardation), rather than the adoption of a gender-biased fashion. Of course the numbers are far too small

to do more than speculate. However, 'the mere dabbler was warned against using electricity', it seems, and the randomly sparse employment of such treatment at Ticehurst points to the Newingtons perhaps not heeding such warnings. It may be more appropriate to view such local experiments as part of the asylum doctors' need 'to establish their professional credentials and social standing, with the general public, and with their medical colleagues in other specialties' (Beveridge & Renvoize, 1988). The failure to take such treatment to the point of inducing a fit – as in modern ECT – should also not be forgotten. Interest in electric therapy declined in the 1890s because of disappointing results and perhaps because the notion of shocking patients was too troubling even for the most hardened Victorian psychiatrist.

(iv) Sedative drugs

As illustrated in Table 12, sedatives became a regular part of treatment at Ticehurst. The two chosen for focus, *Cannabis indica* and chloral represent standard therapy for their time, aimed at quietening restless patients and inducing sleep. Their usage showed no clear relationship to diagnosis, contemporary or modern, and if anything was more hesitant than one might predict given the behavioural disturbances of the clientele. Such suspicion of drug therapy seems in accord with contemporary debates and coherent with a philosophy based on high staff levels and structured physical and 'moral' care.

Cannabis indica (Indian hemp) was described as the 'new toy' in 1858 (Bucknill & Tuke, p. 473), but by 1874 it was regarded (quoting Clouston's Fothergillian Prize Essay for 1870), when mixed with bromide of potassium, as 'more powerful to allay such excitement than any of the other drugs or stimulants tried' (p. 740). Tuke's *Dictionary* (1892) stated that '*Cannabis indica* has been much employed as a hypnotic and as a sedative', quoting Dr Russell Reynolds' advice as to its value in 'senile insomnia', while warning that it was 'of no use in acute mania' (p. 1144). The combination with bromide was endorsed, as it was by Maudsley (1895), 'with the view...of abating it [excitement] by moderate doses without doing harm' (p. 557). Even in 1904 Clouston still reckoned the combination 'one of the best sedatives', while admitting that 'few men have had to treat

Table 12. *The use of* (a) *cannabis* (*Indian hemp*) *and* (b) *chloral preparations at Ticehurst,*
1860–1890 (*selected cases*)

Case no.	Date used	Age	Sex	Marital status	Length of stay (months)	V/R†	Outcome‡	Diagnosis§ Contemporary	Diagnosis§ Modern	Additional treatments
							(a) Cannabis			
186	1867	24	F	S	144	V	Not improved, Asm	Delusions	Schizophrenia (probable)	Mustard bath, stomach pump
216	1867	82	F	W	18	—	Not improved, Asm	Hallucinations delusions	Schizophrenia	Chlorodyne
447	1881	56	F	M	7	V	Removed Dr H.	Melancholia	Major depression	Opium, bromide, shower, bath
450	1881	61	M	M	3	—	Relieved	Melancholia	Major depression (probable)	—
556	1887	35	M	S	9	—	Recovered	Subacute mania	Mania	Hypnotics, enema
557	1887	30	F	S	6	—	Recovered	Acute mania	Mania	Liq. morphii, ice pack (to head)
							(b) Chloral			
274	1870	29	F	S	6	R	Recovered	Delusions	Mania	Mustard, stomach tube
281	1871	38	F	S	4	—	Not improved, Asm	Delusions	Major depression (probable)	Mustard, blister to neck
298	1872	22	M	S	5	—	Recovered	Acute mania with delusions	Mania	Mustard, bromide
329	1874	20	F	S	14	V	Recovered	Acute mania with delusions	Mania	Mustard, bromide stomach tube
392	1878	28	F	S	3	V	Recovered	Mania	Mania	Lotio alum
404	1879	54	F	W	5	—	(Recovered)	Melancholia	(Hypomania)	—
406	1879	54	F	W	24	V	Relieved	Melancholia with delusions	(Schizoaffective)	—

* Female 9, male 3, † Violence and restraint.   ‡ Not improved 4, relieved 2. Asm, transferred to another asylum.   § Schizophrenia
2, manic depressive 9.

diseases for forty years who are not at the end of the time more sceptical about drug treatment and more inclined to trust to the vis medicatrix' (pp. 718–719). While detailed studies of the history of treatment with *Cannabis indica* are not available, evidence from The Retreat's Casebooks (Renvoize & Beveridge, 1989) and those of Chiswick House Asylum (Western MSS in Wellcome Institute) document its general usage in those institutions in the 1880s. Carlson (1974) has suggested that the lack of a standardized preparation and a 'debate about its dangers' led to its gradual disuse in the 1890s.

Chloral shows a similar pattern, although here a more controversial note creeps in. Dr John Campbell (1872) compared single doses of chloral, tincture of Hyoscyamus and bromide in cases of 'Maniacal Excitement' and concluded that chloral was 'the most certain sleep-producer' and acted more quickly than Hyoscyamus. In 1874 Bucknill & Tuke devoted six pages (pp. 730–736) to this 'new narcotic to

which certainly the objection cannot be made that it is inefficacious', but asserted that 'the real value of chloral has not yet been actually determined'. Despite 'its efficacy in producing sleep, it does not tend to cure or even to shorten any form of mental disease', yet 'its value as a temporising remedy must be admitted to be very considerable' (p. 734). Physical side-effects were noted however, and by 1892 (Tuke's *Dictionary*) concern was being expressed as to the need for caution 'in low states of vitality' and the problem of a 'chloral habit or craving' being 'rather easily established' (p. 1135). However, Savage (1891) stated 'I, personally, do not like chloral in these cases [acute manias]…it has a tendency to make patients, who are still taking their food, suspicious and inclined to refuse it' (p. 98). By 1904 Clouston could write: 'Chloral I once believed in far more strongly than I do now…the prolonged use…in some cases certainly tends towards thinness, toward a haggard look in the morning, and toward diminished mental inhibition, as shown by a habit and craving for its use' (p. 712).

Other Casebook material already cited (e.g. Finnane, 1981; Garton, 1988; Renvoize & Beveridge, 1989; the Chiswick House Casebooks) provides supportive evidence of the widespread use of chloral as a sedative in the 1870s and 1880s. But Kirkbride, at The Pennsylvania Hospital (Tomes, 1984, p. 196), 'remained skeptical of claims concerning its superiority over morphine'. Agreeing that 'chloral induced sleep without side effects', he became 'exceedingly cautious in its use' after several 'unexpected deaths'. At The Retreat chloral was used during the 1870s and 1880s 'on an extensive scale', with a marked rise in its usage for 'excitement' (Digby, 1985, p. 129). However, one patient considered it was used to 'quench the poor sufferers into silence', and Digby quotes from the 1877 Select Committee on Lunacy Law, wherein concern as to 'chemical restraint' was raised. At the Utica asylum, by contrast (Dwyer, 1987, p. 123), the superintendent, John Gray, although a keen supporter of chloral therapy, actually 'opposed the substitution of drugs for mechanical restraint'. The Ticehurst material, while confirming the lack of any specific diagnosis (contemporary or modern) related to chloral use, adds little to all this; however, the exhibition of combined treatments (drugs together or with mustard baths, extra nutrition, etc.) in a very disturbed cohort points to the inescapable fact that 'maniacal excitement' invoked desperate remedies. Critics of such therapy, whether they be MPs of 1877 or social historians of the 1980s, have rarely worked in close contact with such patients. As Brown (1982) pointed out in a review of *Museums of Madness* (Scull, 1979), 'no detailed statistical analysis of the patient population of even one major asylum' was attempted, nor were 'the financial ledgers or ward books' examined to support generalizations about drug therapy and diet.

Conclusion

It has been stated (Ray, 1981) that 'it is possible now to get a clearer view of the relationship between the text-book constructions of inmates and asylum practice'. One might suggest that casebook material such as that provided by Ticehurst House adds another level of magnification to the perspective. In fact, the descriptive, diagnostic and therapeutic data that can be drawn from these unique sources makes it imperative that an active policy of locating, collating and preserving such records be initiated at once. The need to limit my enquiries to a primarily diagnostic assessment hides numerous projects of research potential (e.g. therapeutics, language, the role of the physician). Such a focus as mine, employing retrospective diagnoses, nevertheless seemed essential as an initial means of translating nineteenth-century discourses into a modern understanding. As emphasized in the Introduction, this was not done in a spirit of Whiggism or in the belief that modern RDC diagnoses are more valid. It was done to test the social mutability of mental illness as madness, the degree to which the form of such disorder may have been moulded by contemporary experience (e.g. 'taking fright at the Great Exhibition' or 'pressure of business') and inappropriately labelled by the attending physicians. Problems of aetiology, so abundant in many critiques, were therefore negated and have not been discussed. Likewise the effectiveness of 'cures' – as opposed to the straightforward business of care and management – was not deemed important. The routine essentials of behaviour, language and symptoms, in those certified as man, were the business in hand.

Within that context the findings seem incontrovertible. There is a state of being, which can be recognized for at least a century and a half, that constitutes a mental illness. Its most distinctive forms are those now termed 'schizophrenia' and 'manic-depressive' psychosis. These are broad church categories, syndromes rather than single diseases, representative of a Darwinian evolution as much as of a fixed Linnaean classification.

Thus their presentation, behavioural manifestations, ideational content and prevalence probably respond to the longer swell of genetic and environmental change. But at the heart of these conditions is a sameness, a form of symptoms independent of the transitions of society. The severity and physicality of such disorders, complicated as they were in Victorian England by GPI, infectious disease, nutritional and toxic factors, may contrast with modern versions, but do not alter the core of similarity. The contemporary response to their management may therefore be better understood as a vulgar necessity, the inevitable outcome of their continued presence despite the change and apparent progress to an urban industrialism. We need invoke no new illnesses nor restrictive, less accepting, social attitudes. On the contrary, those deemed 'insane' may represent a consistency of behaviour that is relatively surprising given the various social, physical and psychological forces acting on them.

Of course, the Casebooks themselves portray more than just a formal, psychiatric, description. The very process of filling them in seems to have created a change in the understanding of mental illness. From the brevities of terms such as 'delusions' and 'fits of excitement', or even 'occasional paroxysms of insanity', there is a structured expansion to a standard presenting description. An overall term, such as 'mental enfeeblement' or 'mental exaltation', may precede a brief outline of the patient's appearance, speech and style of answering. Comments on the contents of thought – 'suicidal thoughts' or 'delusions...ideas about spirits in the walls' – and memory can be enmeshed in adjectives that report on the mood state. 'Cheerful', 'lively' and 'silly' are used alongside more technical terms such as 'hypochondriacal' or 'depression'.

Yet this linguistic work of description really called for the skills of a novelist, not the stolid conversational tone of practical physicians. Forced by the demands of the 1845 Act into a detailed and repetitive account of lunatic behaviour, alienists soon became exhausted of terminology. It is difficult to imagine a comparable task to that of the daily, or even weekly, reporting of meaningless habits, eccentric activity, incoherent speech and moods too extreme for empathy or too shallow to grasp. The more they wrote, it seems, the less they could connect. Although providing suitable details and material for the scrutiny of Lunacy Commissioners, the process does not seem to have created a psychological language or clarified their diagnoses. Which is not to say that they were unaware of this, that descriptions were not more rounded, or that more sophisticated writing could not emerge. Apart from the prolixities of their admired contemporary, Henry Maudsley, there is much to admire, as Aubrey Lewis (1951) suggested, in some of the regular contributions to the *Journal of Mental Science*. In 1897, for example, Hayes Newington wrote a thoughtful piece on 'Some Mental Aspects of Music' (1897), in which he noted that 'language itself, whether written or spoken, is the necessary precursor of all enquiry and observation...and is not only useful but essential to the powers of cognition and subsequent naming for exchange of ideas'. yet he had to admit, at the end of the article, that 'In my own practice I have met with more than one case in which forecasts, which events have justified, have been made from the results of musical introspection. The tongue can distort or conceal evidences of mental want or of mental preservation which can be revealed with more truthfulness by the fingers or larynx' (p. 721). The inadequacy of their language, whether diagnostic, prognostic, or aetiological, was a significant discovery of the later Victorian psychiatrists. Preventing its degenerating into an absurd pessimism led to their clinging to the ordinary with considerable zeal.

Nevertheless, they were charged with making sense of the management, moral and physical, of mentally ill people. They watched, and wrote as they watched, the course of illnesses. They had to balance out recovery with chronicity, and probably saw what we now call 'tardive dyskinesia' develop in the long-stay patients. But the regular relationship between physical signs and psychotic symptoms – so startlingly obvious in GPI – would have left no room, I suggest, for dualist theories or even for much time spent considering them. The trade in lunacy was self-evidently medical, and the limited evidence we

have of medical attitudes towards lunatics suggests that, by and large, medical men stepped reluctantly, sideways on, into the embarrassing discomforts of caring for the newly corralled insane. The stigma attached to being a 'mad-doctor' was reflected by their portrayal in popular novels such as *Valentine Vox* (Cockton, 1854) and *Hard Cash* (Reade, 1863) and the constant depredations of groups such as the Alleged Lunatic's Friends Society (Hervey, 1986). There was a small cadre of more enthusiastic private asylum keepers, their numbers diminishing as the century progressed. By identifying a recoverable group of patients – now known as 'manic-depressives', but then suffering variably from 'acute mania' or 'melancholia' or whatever – they could maintain a façade of treatment activity that seemed worth while despite the organicity of presentation. The changes noted by Shepherd (1957) in the 1940s seem to be secondary to a similar diagnostic group.

As Hare (1981) has suggested, 'during much of the nineteenth century insanities did tend to dementia. But as the general health of the population gradually improved, this tendency became less; and the effect of this was first apparent in the group of affective disorders, so allowing their identification late in the century as a distinct, non-dementing group.' Given the wealth and social class of the Ticehurst clientele, it is likely that such a distinct group would have here emerged earlier from the fog of general insanity than in the pauper asylums. This treatable form of psychosis thus became the *raison d'être* of the asylum (as seems to have occurred at The Retreat with 'remittant mania' – Digby, 1985, p. 234), its delusions and hallucinations and violence and masturbation intrinsic to an accepted notion of madness. By contrast, the spreading psychiatric involvement in the softer conditions, such as hysteria or the neuroses, was not so appropriate to the place. Such states demanded a subtler language, such as the modern certainties of office neurology or the psycho-economics invented by Sigmund Freud. Hayes Newington certainly talked to his patients, and played music with them, as well as golf and cricket. But his very success in obtaining recoveries, achieved as it was by a considerable cost in personnel and physical effort, seems to have limited his nosological or theoretical vision.

Selecting patients suitable for his regime, narrowing the focus, was the essence of his expertise.

Furthermore, the ambience of Ticehurst was very much behavioural. 'Schizophrenia' conducted itself as a motor disorder as much as a disorder of perception or thinking. Suicide hovered in the wings, violence was a humdrum event. Unpardonable sins, imaginary voices, thoughts being interfered with, mesmeric influences, these were everywhere behind the strange gestures, the masturbatory antics, the bizarre forms of dress, the forced feeding and the mustard baths. Did the hunting and the picnics really assist the dilemma of the mad? Or were they more a means of protecting the carers – the attendants, companions, servants and medical officers – from being driven round the bend by the nature of their task? Distancing themselves by such means from their incomprehensible patients, the Newingtons at least seem to have stayed the course, writing their notes, organizing activities, trying out treatments, keeping up the show, playing in the band.

While the records of Ticehurst House are a rich primary source of historical data, their limits are less easy to define. Ticehurst was a private 'mecca', receiving privileged patients under financial terms that have yet to be clearly unravelled. As stated earlier, it is difficult to place such inmates in a hierarchy of violent or difficult behaviours, since the proprietors had much more control than those in public asylums over both the balance of the clientele and the individual staff/patient ratios. Yet it does provide a kind of time-machine whereby we can observe in formalized, eerie detail the apparent psychopathology of the time. Madness at Ticehurst does not seem to have been, in Foucault's (1967) term, 'a combination of persuasion and mystification' (p. 276). If anything, it was a focus of refusal amid clarification. The Victorian alienists found out just how powerless they were. Battering away at lifelong states, that had never been so faithfully recorded in such negative detail, they paraded a welter of normal staff and comfortable accoutrements. Hearing their imaginary voices, one wishes we could even do half as much.

In the same essay, on music, quoted above, Hayes Newington described:

A case under my care that tells the same tale from day to day. The patient plays on the violoncello and I play on the piano. He is a scholarly musician, with a nice sense of the art of music and with fair execution. He is the subject or urgent aural hallucinations with advancing dementia, which is making its mark alike on musical and general intellect. The 'voices' frequently address him when playing, and I can at once recognise the fact by his withdrawal of intention and feeling, though he goes on playing in an abstracted manner pretty correctly. It is then a question whether the voice or the music is to get the better of him; if the latter he resumes his previous feeling, but if the former he suddenly stops after playing several bars in perfunctory manner. A violent conversation with the voices may put an end to the performance, but a few notes of the piano may bring him back (p. 713).

Bringing back a notion of the world of private asylums will take more than a perfunctory reading of these Casebooks, but they perhaps make it possible for us to be in tune with those times.

Appendix: Some representative cases, 1860–1869

CASE HISTORIES WITH DIAGNOSTIC DISCUSSION AND MODERN (RDC) DIAGNOSIS

1. Case No. 132 Eliza Gipps, schizophrenia (definite).
2. Case No. 223 William Cotton, mania (MD).
3. Case No. 185 Mary Harvey, indefinite (?).
4. Case No. 179 Revd Alexander Black, organic (GPI).
5. Case No. 227 Dr Robert Martin, schizophrenia (paranoid).

1. Patient No. 132 from Casebook 5

Mrs Eliza Gipps, admitted 10. 4. 60, *died* 20. 3. 69 of 'bronchitis'. On admission aged forty, married.

Physical state on admission

'Full habit and lymphatic temperament, eyes suffused and rather weak...head small...melancholy expression of countenance...vascular system weak...respiratory system satisfactory...liver torpid...bowels sluggish...pulse slow and deep seated – tongue rather coated. Skin natural...hands and feet much swollen.'

Mental state

'First symptoms of insanity after her first confinement...very violent and suicidal...to asylum... Langton Hall in Edinburgh...recovered...to the house of a medical man...to home and attendant. Has lately been more impressed with delusions... obstinate in disposition. Very dirty in her habits, voiding her urine about the house and soiling her linen with faeces. She believes there is still the same connection between herself and her child that existed in the womb...that he is influenced by her own state of health, by the food she takes and by the action of her own bodily functions, i.e. if the child goes away she will eat immoderately that he may be supported through her during his absence...She also believes when obeying the call of nature she is passing out her own and the child's life and therefore restrains bowels as long as she can possibly do so...She states that attendants and servants have the power of taking her mind from her, that they can produce internal pain with her pleasure, that they are the cause of her hair falling off, of weakness in the hand, deformity of her toes, etc.'

'She is very suspicious...talks to herself...laughs unmeaningly...desultory in her occupations – seems lost at times and cannot keep up a connection of ideas...Her temper much changed for the worse...at night she is continually getting out of bed...sitting in a chair without occupation of mind or body. Memory and understanding have failed.'

Past history

Active...travelled even widely in Egypt. No family history.

Casebook notes

17. 4. 60 'Unhappy at being separated from her boy...very dirty in her habits...now clean. Takes her meals properly...exercises plentifully...mixing with others.' *23. 4. 60* 'Behaves very well...much lost at times – incapable of keeping up conversation...sleeps better....' *10.5.60* 'Given up dirty habits...very tractable...employs herself in needlework, etc.' *30. 5. 60* '...but requires much attention... melancholy expressing much anxiety about her child...very lost at times and laughs unmeaningly... her answers to questions are irrelevant to the subject and unconnected.' *27. 6. 60* '...delusions that when relieved [of her bowels] she loses a portion of vital power which...injures him and is gradually destroying his life.' [This leads to retention of faeces.] *10. 7. 60* 'A propensity to steal food and in this manner we are able to administer medicine...it is generally put in a fruit tart which is placed aside in the room by the servant, as if she intended it for herself....' *17. 8. 60* '...her ideas are very largely unconnected...unable to keep up conversation with her husband...laughs unmeaningly.' *8. 9. 60* 'More troublesome about food and bowels...in and out of bed at night...sleeping little after 2.0 a.m....requires two persons to be in the room with her...exercises much...attends chapel... but during the service she will sit when she should stand and kneel when it is customary to sit...much lost and quite incapable of collecting or connecting her ideas.' *10. 10. 60* 'Would be very dirty if not closely watched and attended to, obstinate...would stand still and go in the opposite direction from the one he wished...cried excessively.' *31. 12. 60* 'Does not improve in mental condition...her habits are better...constantly asked about her child. *2. 2. 61* 'Same.' *22. 5. 61* 'Her intellect becomes weaker...she laughs involuntarily a great deal and talks unconnectedly...unable to fix herself steadily to any employment. Bodily health good.' *17. 9. 61* 'irritable and excited lately – has lashed out and tried to scratch or squeeze their throats – very spiteful – no affection for her husband...makes strange howling noises at times.' [From now on the notes are largely 'the same' or 'no change'.] *25. 3. 66* 'Robust bodily health, as demented as hitherto...less liable to hysterical paroxysms. Retains her delusions.' *30. 6. 67* 'Her letters are as incoherent and jumbled as her language...[the inserted letter shows gross thought disorder]...rarely does work....' *31. 12. 67* 'Lies for hours in a dreamy vacant way, in one attitude, on the sofa. Sometimes laughs and chatters in a meaningless way. Bodily health very good.' *June 1868* 'Occasional paroxysms of rage...attacks her attendant savagely.' *23. 3. 69* 'Died of bronchitis secondary to? "typhoid character".'

This case was diagnosed as RDC 'schizophrenia', definite, on the grounds of her bizarre delusions about her child and body, the evidence of thought withdrawal [attendants having the power of taking her mind from her], persistent descriptions of formal thought-disorder, and evidence of negativism ['she would stand still and go in an opposite direction from the one he wished'].

2. Patient No. 223 from Casebook 13

William Henry Cotton, admitted 15. 5. 67, discharged 5. 7. 68 as 'unimproved'. Described as fifty-four, single and a vicar who had been ten years in his living.

Physical state on admission

'Corpulent'...head described as 'large and regular in formation though somewhat sloping anteriorly but expanding naturally'. Features 'massive and pronounced and pregnant with intelligence and energy'.

Past history

'Eccentric'...scholar of Eton and a first at Oxford. In 1847 suffered from 'brain fever' on return from New Zealand and in 1857 described as 'excited/restless'.

Present illness

Transferred from Manor House, Chiswick, where he had been since May 1866. [Dr Tuke.] He had an affair there with a maid called Nellie. His certificates described him as 'incoherent, excited, and (making?) irrelevant conversation. Strangely connected and disordered account concerning money, etc. Spending money faster than he received it...large debts...up and about almost all night'.

Mental state

'Great intellectual acuteness and excellent memory. Untidy and slovenly. Conversation rational, no paralysis. Disposition wilful, temper fickle and hasty.' No delusions or hallucinations 'so far'.

Casebook notes

'He writes long letters...want of fixity and steadiness...*outré* execution upon the keyboard... multifarious occupations.' He is described as 'untidy', 'unclean', with 'purposeless way', and as being 'unable to stick to one job'. His clothes are strange and disordered, he suffers from violent outbursts, is excited, flirting with kitchen maids, escaped twice, writing verses, impulsive and mercurial, jovial and happy. A special nurse is employed. On *29. 2. 68* a Dr L. Robertson diagnosed him as 'cured' from intellectual disorder, but he now laboured under a disorder of 'an affected line', in fact 'moral insanity'. Dr Robertson therefore recommended removal from the asylum and he was discharged 'unimproved'.

Diagnosis

In view of the descriptions of Mr Cotton as distractible, constantly on the go, spending money and writing letters, not sleeping appropriately, as well as his 'strangely connected and disordered accounts' (which may represent 'flight of ideas'), the diagnosis of 'mania' seems acceptable according to RDC standards. The interesting contemporary diagnosis, after his prolonged admission, of 'moral insanity', reflects on the vague usage of this latter term.

3. Patient No. 185 from Casebook 10

Miss Mary Harvey. Admitted 22. 11. 64 and discharged 22. 6. 67 as 'unimproved'. She is described as a sixty-year-old gentlewoman, unmarried. There are brief physical details describing her as having a neurosanguine temperament, her head as normal and her eyes as looking down. She has been for the previous eight years under Dr Sutherland's care.

Mental state

'Temper sharp and petulant, slaps at people. She walks incessantly up and down the room. Refusing to answer questions, telling you "to be banned" or "you cannot make me young again". No evidence of general paralysis or epilepsy. Not dangerous to others, not suicidal.' The case is quoted as 'crossed in love'.

Casebook notes

29. 11. 64 'Slaps her attendant...uses bad language...in the habit of taking morphine at night, but none now. Less excitable.' *5. 12. 65* 'More calm...sits in the armchair generally with eyes shut...now appears to pay attention...sleeps well.' *12. 12. 64* 'Amenable to instructions...fond of listening to the organ.' [Entries then are 'as usual', or 'bad language' until March 1866] – 'Unaltered in body and mind'. 'Takes regular exercise.' *31. 3. 67* 'Never seems to smile...often in her chair with her fingers applied to her mouth and stuck up her nostrils ...ill condition generally...avoids all treatment and interference.' *20. 2. 67* 'Removed unimproved.'

Diagnosis

Apart from odd behaviours and evidence of a movement/posture disorder, which may be catatonic or may be an indication of negativism, nothing in the notes is sufficient to supply a diagnosis. Miss Harvey is therefore categorized as 'indefinite' and is quite typical of the chronic type of case that comes through and often stays in the asylum for many years.

4. Patient No. 179 from Casebook 10

Reverend Alexander Black. Admitted 2.8.64 and died 26.12.65. Described as a fifty-two-year-old single man. A clerk in holy orders of the established church.

Physical state on admission

'Neurosanguinous temperament. Countenance is somewhat fatuitous. Idiotic kind of smile frequently present. Head is fair sized and forehead slightly overlapping.' (No other evidence of physical abnormality is noted.)

History of present illness

'This has gradually been coming on for the last year or so. He has become very childish. At billiards each time he is asking which is his ball...playing cricket in the afternoon...is asking the next morning whether he ever played cricket here. Evinces great loss of memory. Constantly talking at every available opportunity in an exalted strain, e.g. repeating at length a long account of the French war in Russia. His memory and understanding are impaired. Unquestionably symptoms of general paralysis. Tremulous movements of tongue. Defective articulation... clipping his words, e.g. arch for architecture. Gait weak and unsteady (has been an itinerant feature...in France and every county in England).'

Casebook notes

6. 8. 64 'Settled quietly...constantly wandering about looking for his hat and stick. Cannot find his own room when he has come out. Talks in a loud idiotic manner...repeating the same stories...mumbling and clipping his words. Laughing and replies 'what' three or four times when asked a question. Not able apparently to understand it.' *10. 8. 64* 'Appetite moderate...sleeps fairly...reads...cricket...attends concerts.' *13. 8. 64* 'Untidy in dress...straggling gait. Will not allow barber to shave him...repeats the same stories.' *20. 8. 64* 'Attempts to run away...does not appear to have any decided object to get to anywhere particularly.' *6. 9 . 64* 'Very fidgetty and excitable...imagines he has some food corruption in his stomach...makes himself sick...aspect more haggard and pale.' *1. 10. 64* 'Speech is very thick...wagging his head from side to side...makes water in the coal bucket but then denies it. Talking at length of lost property.' *16. 11. 64* 'Cannot understand anything [therefore no use attending prayers]'. *5. 1. 65* 'More imbecile and lost. Grinds his teeth occasionally.' *23. 1. 65* 'Can scarcely understand anything except by signs...very obstinate.' *28. 2. 65* 'Very noisy...refuses food frequently...wets the bed.' *21. 3. 65* 'Very noisy...saying "my yahs"...' *'Visited by brother, did not recognise him. Allows saliva to run out of the sides of his mouth.' *29. 4. 65* 'Very imbecile and noisy when out walking.' *25. 5. 65* 'Partial paralysis of left side...recovered. Very noisy, appetite good, walks out daily.' *10. 7. 65* 'The same...answers "yes" to everything.' *16. 8. 65* 'Stumbles about if left by himself...' *11. 9. 65* 'Very demented.' *5. 12. 65* 'Manifestly weaker...bed sores...swallows with extreme difficulty...'. *26. 12. 65* 'Died of general paralysis.'

Diagnosis

The description of physical decline, associated with neurological symptoms and memory impairment, is clearly indicative of an organic illness, most likely general paralysis of the insane. The Reverend Black is much less violent and grandiose than many of the more colourful general paralytics, but he illustrates well the decline into idiocy and the increasing neurological impairment. A number of these cases suffer from increasing fits as well.

5. Patient No. 227 from Casebook 13

Robert Martin. Admitted 21. 9. 67, discharged 24. 12. 68 as 'recovered'. Described as forty, single MD from Cambridge and a physician on the staff at St Bartholomew's Hospital. He was transferred from Haddon Place Asylum in Hertfordshire, where he had been for three months under the care of a Dr Smith.

Physical state on admission

'Pale and careworn...large circular head, rather flat superiorly and expanded laterally. Denuded of hair on top.'

Mental state

'Affable...cheerful...memory intact.' Gait and articulation are reported as normal. He is described as preoccupied with an 'unmistakable watchfulness'. No paralysis or epilepsy.

History of present illness

'First illness lasting for some five months. However, his conduct has been strange and altered for several years. Suspecting servants of conspiracy against him...informing the police.' Became violent, and strange treatment of a man-servant led to him being so frightened that he escaped by the roof. The certificates state 'persons are lying in wait to accuse him of grave crimes' and 'victim of a conspiracy' as well as 'constant restlessness' and 'an idea that people are moving about his rooms all night to implicate him in some improper action'.

Casebook notes [undated]

'Conspiracy notions...guarded and argumentative in his manner and language and a peculiar sensitiveness and suspiciousness.' 'Hints' given him that had revealed the 'myth' of his existence. He complains of sleeping badly 'due to tension and something else which he does not define'. His health and spirits and rational pursuits are noted. He is described as 'gathering hidden meanings' from 'jargon and odd speeches of other patients'. 'He seriously believes other patients are prompted or "primed" to say things before him, to apply "tests" in this way. He says that he heard London's street boys calling out his name and singing about him...that women were made to follow him into his house...daily expectation of some serious mischief arising here...he intimated that the Queen is in possession of his story [agitated]...dread of a "charge" being brought against him...a coterie exists in the house co-operating with the parties out of doors...conspiracy, ramifications of which are deeply fixed in society through the influence of Freemasons, Oddfellows, Licensed Victuallers and Horse Guards. He is constantly discovering fresh indications and manifestations of these.' *31. 1. 68* He finds hints constantly in 'agony columns' of newspapers. These are telling how to act, etc.

Described as 'monomania'...in other respects 'clever, intelligent, rational, amiable, honourable and gentlemanlike'. He says that he is 'inconveniently sane' and it is 'better to be strangled than to be in an asylum all one's days'...he searches the papers daily for 'advertisements [with great eagerness] that may refer to him'...he has suspicions of strangers, these become less so. On *6. 11. 68* he goes out on probation and on *28. 12. 68* is discharged as 'recovered'.

Diagnosis

In view of his delusional ideas, of a paranoid nature, with marked ideas of reference and likely hallucinations [hearing London street boys calling out his name] this man was diagnosed as having 'paranoid schizophrenia'. The lack of details or any significant improvement in his mental state may be related to the fact that he is a physician. The use of the term 'recovered' here is doubtful, to say the least.

REFERENCES

Acheson, D. (1985). That over-used word Community. *Health Trends* **17**, 3.

Alexander, F. & Selesnick, S. (1966). *The History of Psychiatry.* Harper and Row: New York.

Allderidge, P. (1985). Bedlam: fact or fantasy? In *The Anatomy of Madness*, vol. 1 (ed. W. Bynum, R. Porter and M. Shepherd), pp. 17–33. Tavistock: London.

American Psychiatric Association (1980). *Diagnostic and Statistical Manual of Mental Disorders*, 3rd edn. APA: Washington, DC.

Anderson, O. (1988). *Suicide in Victorian and Edwardian England.* Clarendon Press: Oxford.

Barton, R. (1976). *Institutional Neurosis* (3rd edn). John Wright: Bristol.

Bayle, A. L. J. (1856). *Traité des Malaides du Cervaux et de ses Membranes.* Gabon: Paris.

Berrios, G. E. (1984). Descriptive psychopathology: conceptual and historical aspects. *Psychological Medicine* **14**, 303–313.

Berrios, G. E. (1988). Melancholia and depression during the 19th century: a conceptual history. *British Journal of Psychiatry* **153**, 298–304.

Berson, R. J. (1983). Capgras' syndrome. *American Journal of Psychiatry* **140**, 969–978.

Bevan Lewis, W. (1890). *A Textbook of Mental Diseases.* P. Blakiston, Son and Co.: Philadelphia.

Beveridge, A. W. & Renvoize, E. B. (1988). Electricity: a history of its use in the treatment of mental illness in Britain during the second half of the 19th century. *British Journal of Psychiatry* **153**, 157–162.

Bleuler, E. (1950). *Dementia Praecox or the Group of Schizophrenias* (translated from 1911 edn. by J. Zinkin). International Universities Press: New York.

Brown, E. M. (1985). 'What shall we do with the inebriate?' Asylum treatment and the disease concept of alcoholism in the late nineteenth century. *Journal of the History of Behavioral Sciences* **21**, 48–59.

Brown, T. E. (1982). The mental hospital and its historians. An essay review. *Bulletin of the History of Medicine* **56**, 109–114.

Bucknill, J. C. & Tuke, D. H. (1858). *A Manual of Psychological Medicine.* John Churchill: London. (Facsimile edition 1968, Hafner: New York and London.)

Bucknill, J. C. & Tuke, D. H. (1874). *A Manual of Psychological Medicine.* John Churchill: London.

Busfield, J. (1986). *Managing Madness: Changing Ideas and Practice.* Hutchinson: London.

Bynum, W. F., Porter, R. & Shepherd, M. (1985). Introduction to *The Anatomy of Madness*. Vol. I. People and Ideas (pp. 1–24). Vol. II: Institutions and Society (pp. 1–16). Tavistock: London.

Bynum, W. F., Porter, R. & Shepherd, M. (1988). Introduction to *The Anatomy of Madness*. Vol. III. The Asylum and its Psychiatry (pp. 1–12). Routledge: London.

Campbell, J. (1872). On the relative efficacy of tincture of Hyoscyamus. bromide of potassium, and chloral, in single doses, on maniacal excitement. *Journal of Mental Science* **17**, 519–525.

Carlson, E. T. (1974). Cannabis indica in 19th-century psychiatry. *American Journal of Psychiatry* **131**, 1004–1007.

Cheyne, G. (1733). *The English Malady: or a Treatise of Nervous Diseases of All Kinds, as Spleen, Vapours, Lowness of Spirits, Hypochondriacal, and Hysterical Distempers etc.* Strahan and Leake: London.

Clark, M. J. (1981). The rejection of psychological approaches to mental disorder in late nineteenth-century British psychiatry. In *Madhouses, Mad-Doctors and Madmen* (ed. A. Scull), pp. 271–312. Athlone Press: London.

Clark, M. J. (1983). 'A plastic power ministering to organisation': interpretations of the mind–body relation in late nineteenth-century British psychiatry. *Psychological Medicine* **13**, 487–497.

Clark, M. J. (1988). 'Morbid Introspection' – unsoundness of mind, and British psychological medicine c. 1830–c. 1900. In *The Anatomy of Madness*. Vol. III. *The Asylum and its Psychiatry* (ed. W. Bynum, R. Porter and M. Shepherd), pp. 71–101. Routledge: London.

Clouston, T. S. (1871). The Action of Neurotic Medicines in Insanity: being 'Observations and Experiments on the Use of Opium, Bromide of Potassium, and Cannabis Indica in Insanity, 'especially in regard to the effects of the two latter given separately.' The Fothergillian Prize Essay for 1870. *Journal of Mental Science* **17**, 278–285.

Clouston, T. S. (1887). *How Pleasant Surroundings and Conditions Affect the Health and Happiness.* MacNiven and Wallace, Edinburgh Health Society: Edinburgh.

Clouston, T. S. (1888). Presidential address. *Journal of Mental Science* **34**, 325–348.

Clouston, T. S. (1904). *Clinical Lectures on Mental Diseases*, 6th edn. J. and A. Churchill: London.

Cochrane, D. (1988). 'Humane, economical, and medically wise': the L.C.C. as administrators of Victorian lunacy policy. In *The Anatomy of Madness*. Vol. III. *The Asylum and its Psychiatry* (ed. W. Bynum, R. Porter and M. Shepherd), pp. 247–272. Routledge: London.

Cockton, H. (1854). *Valentine Vox – The Ventriloquist.* George Routledge: London.

Colaizzi, J. (1989). *Homicidal Insanity, 1800–1985.* University of Alabama Press: Tuscaloosa and London.

Conolly, J. (1830). *The Indications of Insanity.* John Taylor: London. Reprinted 1964 (ed. R. Hunter and I. Macalpine). Dawsons: London.

Conolly, J. (1847). *The Construction and Government of Lunatic Asylums, and Hospitals for the Insane.* John Churchill: London. Reprinted 1968 (ed. R. Hunter and I. Macalpine). Dawsons: London.

Conolly, J. (1856). *The Treatment of the Insane without Mechanical Restraints.* Smith, Elder and Co: London. Reprinted 1973 (ed. R. Hunter and I. MacAlpine). Dawsons: London.

Cooper, J. and Sartorius, N. (1977). Cultural and temporal variations in schizophrenia: a speculation on the importance of industrialization. *British Journal of Psychiatry* **130**, 50–55.

de Boismont, A. B. (1859). *On Hallucinations* (trans. R. T. Hulme). Henry Renshaw: London.

Defendorf, A. (1902). *Clinical Psychiatry.* Macmillan: London. (See Kraepelin, 1902.)

De Watteville, A. (1885). Practical remarks on the use of electricity in mental disease. *Journal of Mental Science* **30**, 483–488.

Digby, A. (1984). The changing profile of a nineteenth-century asylum: the York Retreat. *Psychological Medicine* **14**, 739–748.

Digby, A. (1985). *Madness, Morality and Medicine. A Study of the York Retreat 1796–1914.* Cambridge University Press: Cambridge.

Discussion (1885). *Journal of Mental Science* **31**, 284–286.

Dwyer, E. (1987). *Homes for the Mad. Life inside Two Nineteenth-Century Asylums.* Rutgers University Press: New Brunswick and London.

Eastwood, J. W. (1863). On private asylums for the insane. *Journal of Mental Science* **9**, 319–327.

Ellis, H. (1900). *Studies in the Psychology of Sex*, vol. 2. F. A. Davis and Co.: Philadelphia.

Enoch, M. D. & Trethowen, W. H. (1979). *Uncommon Psychiatric Syndromes.* John Wright: Bristol.

Esquirol, J. E. D. (1845). *Mental Maladies: A Treatise on Insanity* (trans. E. K. Hunt). Lea and Blanchard: Philadelphia. (Facsimile edition 1965. Hafner: New York.)

Feuchtersleben, E. von. (1847). *The Principles of Medical Psychology*, (trans. H. Evan Lloyd). Sydenham Society: London.

Finnane, M. (1981). *Insanity and the Insane in Post-Famine Ireland.* Croom Helm: London.

Fish, F. (1974). *Fish's Clinical Psychopathology* (ed. Max Hamilton). John Wright and Sons: Bristol.

Foucault, M. (1967). *Madness and Civilization* (trans. R. Howard). Tavistock: London.

Foulds, G. A. (1976). *The Hierarchical Nature of Personal Illness.* Academic Press: London and Orlando.

French Retrospect. (1884). *Journal of Mental Science* 30, 150–151.

Garton, S. (1988). *Medicine and Madness. A Social History of Insanity in New South Wales 1880–1940.* New South Wales University Press: Sydney.

Goffman, E. (1961). *Asylums: Essays on the Social Situation of Mental Patients and Other Inmates.* Anchor Books: Garden City, New York.

Griesinger, W. (1867). *Mental Pathology and Therapeutics* (trans. C. L. Robertson and L. Rutherford). New Sydenham Society: London.

Gull, W. W. (1874). Anorexia nervosa (apepsia hysteria, anorexia hysterica). *Transactions of the Clinical Society of London* 7, 22–28.

Häfner, H. (1987). The concept of disease in psychiatry. *Psychological Medicine* 17, 11–14.

Hare, E. H. (1959). The origin and spread of dementia paralytica. *Journal of Mental Science* 105, 594–626.

Hare, E. H. (1962). Masturbatory insanity: the history of an idea. *Journal of Mental Science* 108, 1–25.

Hare, E. H. (1981). The two manias: a study of the evolution of the modern concept of mania. *British Journal of Psychiatry* 138, 88–99.

Hare, E. H. (1983). Was insanity on the increase? *British Journal of Psychiatry* 142, 439–455.

Hare, E. H. (1986). Aspects of the epidemiology of schizophrenia. *British Journal of Psychiatry* 149, 554–561.

Hare, E. H. (1988). Schizophrenia as a recent disease. *British Journal of Psychiatry* 153, 521–531.

Haslam, J. (1798). *Observations on Insanity.* Rivington: London.

Haslam, J. (1810). *Illustrations of Madness.* Rivington: London. Reprinted 1988 (ed. R. Porter). Routledge: London.

Hervey, N. (1986). Advocating or folly: the alleged Lunatics' Friend Society; 1845–63. *Medical History* 30, 245–275.

Hervey, N. (1987). The Lunacy Commission 1845–60, with special reference to the implementation of policy in Kent and Surrey. 2 vols. Ph.D. Thesis: University of Bristol.

Hill, Gardiner, R. (1838). *Total Abolition of Personal Restraint in the Treatment of the Insane.* A lecture on the management of lunatic asylums and the treatment of the insane. Simpkin, Marshall: London.

Hirsch, S. R. & Shepherd, M. eds. (1974). *Themes and Variations in European Psychiatry.* John Wright and Sons: Bristol.

Hunter, R. & MacAlpine, I. (1963). *Three Hundred Years of Psychiatry 1535–1860.* Oxford University Press: London.

Hunter, R. & MacAlpine, I. (1974). *Psychiatry for the Poor.* Dawsons: London.

Hunter, R., Earl, C. J. & Thornicroft, S. (1964). An apparently irreversible syndrome of abnormal movements following phenothiazine medication. *Proceedings of the Royal Society of Medicine* 57, 758–762.

International Classification of Diseases, Ninth Revision (1978). WHO: Geneva.

James, R. L. & May, P. R. A. (1981). Diagnosing schizophrenia: Professor Kraepelin and the Research Diagnostic Criteria. *American Journal of Psychiatry* 138, 501–504.

Jeste, D. V., del Carmen, R., Lohr, J. B. & Wyatt, R. J. (1985). Did schizophrenia exist before the eighteenth century? *Comprehensive Psychiatry* 26, 493–503.

Johnstone, E. C., Cunningham Owens, D. G., Gold, A., Crow, T. J. & MacMillan, J. F. (1981). Institutionalization and the defects of schizophrenia. *British Journal of Psychiatry* 139, 195–203.

Jones, K. (1982). Scull's dilemma. *British Journal of Psychiatry* 141, 221–226.

Kendell, R. E. (1989). Clinical validity. *Psychological Medicine* 19, 45–55.

Kennedy, P. F., Hershon, H. I. & McGuire, R. J. (1971). Extra-pyramidal disorders after prolonged phenothiazine therapy. *British Journal of Psychiatry* 118, 509–518.

Klaf, F. S. & Hamilton, J. F. (1961). Schizophrenia – a hundred years ago and today. *Journal of Mental Science* 107, 819–827.

Kosky, R. (1986). From mortality to madness: a reappraisal of the asylum movement in psychiatry 1800–1940. *Australian and New Zealand Journal of Psychiatry* 20, 180–187.

Kraepelin, E. (1902). *Clinical Psychiatry.* (Abstracted and adapted from the 6th German edition of 'Lehrbuch Der Psychiatrie' by A. Ross Denfendorf.) Macmillan and Co.: New York.

Kraepelin, E. (1912). *Lectures on Clinical Psychiatry* (ed. T. Johnstone, 3rd edn). Baillière, Tindall and Cox: London.

Kräupl Taylor, F. (1979). *Psychopathology: Its Causes and Symptoms.* Quartermaine House: Sunbury-on-Thames.

Kroll, J. & Bachrach, B. (1982). Medieval visions and contemporary hallucinations. *Psychological Medicine* 12, 709–721.

Lancet (1986). Devils in Disguise. (Editorial) i, 25–26.

Leigh, D. (1961). *The Historical Development of British Psychiatry.* Vol. 1. *18th and 19th Century.* Pergamon Press: London.

Lewis, A. J. (1934). Melancholia: a historical review. *Journal of Mental Science* 80, 1–42.

Lewis, A. J. (1951). Henry Maudsley: his work and influence. *Journal of Mental Science* 97, 259–277.

Lunacy in England and Wales (1910). Supplement to *British Medical Journal* ii, 429–431.

MacAlpine, I. & Hunter, R. (1956). *Schizophrenia 1677. A Psychiatric Study of an Illustrated Autobiographical Record of Demoniacal Possession.* Dawson and Sons: London.

MacKenzie, C. (1985). Social factors in the admission, discharge and continuing stay of patients at Ticehurst Asylum, 1845–1917. In *The Anatomy of Madness* (ed. W. F. Bynum, R. Porter and M. Shepherd), pp. 147–174. Tavistock: London.

MacKenzie, C. (1986). A family asylum: a history of the private madhouse at Ticehurst in Sussex, 1792–1917. Ph.D. thesis: University of London.

MacLeod, R. M. (1967). The edge of hope: social policy and chronic alcoholism 1870–1900. *Journal of the History of Medicine and Allied Sciences* 22, 215–245.

Maudsley, H. (1868). Illustrations of a variety of insanity. *Journal of Mental Science* 14, 149–162.

Maudsley, H. (1895). *The Pathology of Mind.* Macmillan: London. (Reprinted 1979, Julian Friedmann: London.)

Medical Superintendents, The (1901). Some incidents in the history and practice of Ticehurst Asylum. *Journal of Mental Science* 47, 62–72.

Mellor, C. S. (1970). First-rank symptoms of schizophrenia. *British Journal of Psychiatry* 117, 15–23.

Mercier, C. (1902). *A Text-Book of Insanity.* Swan Sonnenschein and Co.: London.

Mullen, P. E. (1986). The mental state and states of mind. In *Essentials of Postgraduate Psychiatry* (ed. P. Hill, R. Murray and A. Thorley), pp. 3–36. Grune and Stratton: London.

Murray, R. (1986). Schizophrenia. In *Essentials of Postgraduate Psychiatry* (ed. P. Hill, R. Murray and A. Thorley), pp. 339–379. Grune and Stratton: London.

Newington, A. S. L. (1865). On a new remedial agent in the treatment of insanity and other diseases. *Lancet* i, 621.

Newington, C. (1826). 'Mr. Newington's instrument for administering food, etc.' *Lancet* i, 845–846.

Newington, H. H. (1874). Mania a Potu. *Edinburgh Medical Journal* 20, 493–500.

Newington, H. H. (1877). Case of an extraordinary number of convulsions in an epileptic patient with remarks on nutrient enemata. *Journal of Mental Science* 23, 89–95.

Newington, H. H. (1885). The abolition of private asylums. *Journal of Mental Science* 31, 138–147.

Newington, H. H. (1887). What are the tests of fitness for discharge from asylums? *Journal of Mental Science* 32, 491–500.

Newington, H. H. (1897). Some mental aspects of music. *Journal of Mental Science* 43, 704–723.

Newington, T. (1879). Feeding by the nose. *Lancet* i, 83.

Obituary (1917). Herbert Francis Hayes Newington, F.R.C.P. Edin., M.R.C.S. Eng. *Journal of Mental Science* **63**, 461–467.

Owens, D. G. C., Johnstone, E. C. & Frith, C. D. (1982). Spontaneous involuntary disorders of movement. *Archives of General Psychiatry* **39**, 452–461.

Parfitt, D. (1985). Asylum 1929. *British Journal of Clinical and Social Psychiatry* **3**, 3–5.

Parry-Jones, W. L. (1972). *The Trade in Lunacy*. Routledge and Kegan Paul: London.

Pinel, P. (1806). *A Treatise on Insanity* (trans. D. D. Davis). Cadell and Davis: London. (Facsimile edition 1962; Hafner: New York.)

Porter, R. (1987). *A Social History of Madness*. Weidenfeld and Nicholson: London.

Ray, L. J. (1981). Models of madness in Victorian asylum practice. *Archives of European Sociology* **22**, 229–264.

Reade, C. (1863). *Hard Cash: A Matter of Fact Romance*. (Serialized in *All the Year Round*, ed. C. Dickens.) Chapman and Hall: London.

Renvoize, E. B. & Beveridge, A. W. (1989). Mental illness and the late Victorians: a study of patients admitted to three asylums in York, 1880–1884. *Psychological Medicine* **19**, 19–28.

Report of the Select Committee on Lunacy Law (1877). HMSO: London.

Robinson, A. D. T. (1988). A century of delusions in South West Scotland. *British Journal of Psychiatry* **153**, 163–167.

Rogers, D. (1985). The motor disorders of severe psychiatric illness: a conflict of paradigms. *British Journal of Psychiatry* **147**, 221–232.

Rothman, D. J. (1971). *The Discovery of the Asylum. Social Order and Disorder in the Early Republic*. Little, Brown: Boston.

Savage, G. (1891). *Insanity and Allied Neuroses*, 3rd edn. Churchill: London.

Scheff, T. J. (1966). *Being Mentally Ill: A Sociological Theory*. Aldine: Chicago.

Scull, A. (1977). *Decarceration: Community Treatment and the Deviant – A Radical View*. Prentice-Hall: Englewood Cliffs, N.J.

Scull, A. (1979). *Museums of Madness*. Allen Lane: London.

Scull, A. (1984). Was insanity increasing? A response to Edward Hare. *British Journal of Psychiatry* **144**, 432–436.

Shepherd, M. (1957). *A Study of the Major Psychoses in an English County*. Maudsley Monographs No. 3. Oxford University Press: London.

Skae, D. (1863). A rational and practical classification of insanity. *Journal of Mental Science* **9**, 309–319.

Showalter, E. (1985). *The Female Malady. Women, Madness and English Culture, 1830–1980*. Pantheon Books: New York.

Spitzer, R., Endicott, J. & Robins, E. (1975). *Research Diagnostic Criteria*. New York State Psychiatric Institute: New York.

Spitzer, R., Endicott, J. & Robins, E. (1978). Research Diagnostic Criteria: rationale and reliability. *Archives of General Psychiatry* **35**, 773–782.

Spitzka, E. C. (1887, 1888). Cases of masturbation (masturbatic insanity). *Journal of Mental Science* **33**, 57–73, 238–254, 395–401; **34**, 52–61, 216–225.

Stahl, S. M. (1986). Tardive dyskinesia: natural history studies assist the pursuit of preventive therapies. *Psychological Medicine* **16**, 491–494.

Sutherland, H. (1883). Prognosis in cases of refusal of food. *Journal of Mental Science* **29**, 178–188.

Sutton, T. (1813). *Tracts on Delirium Tremens*. Underwood: London.

Szasz, T. (1972). *The Myth of Mental Illness*. Paladin: London.

Tomes, N. (1984). *A Generous Confidence. Thomas Story Kirkbride and the Art of Asylum-Keeping 1840–1883*. Cambridge University Press: Cambridge.

Tomes, N. (1988). The great restraint controversy: a comparative perspective on Anglo-American psychiatry in the nineteenth century. In *The Anatomy of Madness*. Vol. III. *The Asylum and its Psychiatry* (ed. W. F. Bynum, R. Porter and M. Shepherd), pp. 190–225. Routledge: London.

Torrey, E. F. (1980). *Schizophrenia and Civilization*. Jason Aronson: New York.

Tsuang, M. T. & Winokur, G. (1975). The Iowa 500: fieldwork in a 35-year follow-up of depression, mania, and schizophrenia. *Canadian Psychiatric Association Journal* **20**, 359–365.

Tuke, D. H. (ed.). (1892). *A Dictionary of Psychological Medicine*, 2 vols. J. and A. Churchill: London.

Tuke, S. (1813). *Description of the Retreat; An Institution near York for Insane Persons of the Society of Friends*. (Facsimile edition 1964, ed. H. Hunter and I. MacAlpine.) Dawsons: London.

Turner, T. H. (1985). The past of psychiatry: why build asylums? *Lancet* ii, 709–711.

Waddington, J. L. (1987). Tardive dyskinesia in schizophrenia and other disorders: associations with ageing, cognitive dysfunction, and structural brain pathology in relation to neuroleptic exposure. *Human Psychopharmacology* **2**, 11–22.

Wing, J. K. (1961). A simple and reliable subclassification of chronic schizophrenia. *Journal of Mental Science* **107**, 862–875.

Wing, J. K. & Brown, G. W. (1970). *Institutionalism and Schizophrenia*. Cambridge University Press: Cambridge.

Wing, J. K., Cooper, J. E. & Sartorius, N. (1974). *Measurement and Classification of Psychiatric Symptoms*. Cambridge University Press: London.

Winslow, F. (1866). *Obscure Diseases of the Brain and Mind*, 2nd American from 3rd revised English edn. Henry Lee: Philadelphia.

Wraxall, Sir F. (1862). De Lunatico, *Temple Bar* **5**, 528–541.

Zilboorg, G. & Henry, G. W. (1941). *A History of Medical Psychology*. W. W. Norton: New York.

Psychological Medicine

Editor
MICHAEL SHEPHERD

Emeritus Professor, Institute of Psychiatry,
University of London

Psychological Medicine publishes original research in clinical psychiatry and the basic sciences related to it. These comprise not only the several fields of biological inquiry traditionally associated with medicine, but also the various psychological and social sciences whose relevance to medicine has become increasingly apparent. Editorials and commissioned review articles are published regularly. The journal also carries an extensive book review section. Periodic supplements to the journal will be published and sent free to subscribers. They may also be purchased separately. The current titles are:

ISSN 0033-2917   ISBN 0 521 42986 2